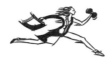

TOO BUSY TO EXERCISE

PORTER SHIMER

A Storey Publishing Book

Storey Communications, Inc.
Schoolhouse Road
Pownal, Vermont 05261

The mission of Storey Communications is to serve our customers by publishing practical information that encourages personal independence in harmony with the environment.

Edited by Pamela Lappies
Cover design by Meredith Maker
Text design by Carol J. Jessop, Black Trout Design
Text production by Faith E. Kaufman, Black Trout Design
Illustrations by Laura Tedeschi
Reviewed by Randi Haskins, licensed Physical Therapist and co-owner of Darshan Physical Therapy, Williamstown, Massachusetts, and Great Barrington, Massachusetts
Indexed by Northwind Editorial Services

Printed in the United States by Quebecor Printing
ISBN 0-88266-936-2

66 No time for jogging
Or going to the gym
For a healthier heart
Or fewer folds of the chin?

Then relax and read this book;
Its message will leave you pleased.
You're too busy to exercise
Only if you're too busy to breathe. **99**

— Porter Shimer

TABLE OF CONTENTS

Acknowledgments

My sincere thanks to Claire Kowalchik for her love and her fax machine;

To Pamela Lappies for her guidance and eleventh-hour insights;

To Randi Haskins, licensed Physical Therapist and co-owner of Darshan Physical Therapy of Williamstown, Massachusetts, and Great Barrington, Massachusetts, for sharing her hands-on knowledge of the human body;

And to my buddy Skip O'Neill for following me to the gas station that night.

A Pep Talk

I know. You're very busy. So I'll be as brief as possible right from the start. I understand your dilemma, because I've experienced it: The harder we work, the softer we seem to get. The reward for working our buns off in this push-button world is a pair of buns we can't work off. And you're right: It's not fair.

With our soft physiques may come some other threats, moreover — things such as blood pressure or cholesterol levels that furrow our doctors' brows. Or levels of stress that have us getting too much exercise reaching into our liquor or medicine cabinets. Or sleep that's become about as restful as a bullfight.

But then who wouldn't become a little frayed? Between our jobs, the commute to and from our jobs, our family duties, and whatever community involvement we can squeeze in, we go nonstop from the second we're rattled awake by our alarms.

Nor do full-time homekeepers have it any easier if anyone between the ages of about six months and six years is included in the mix. Until children finally begin school, it's part of their caretaker's job to be teacher, principal, guidance counselor, physical education instructor, cook, bus driver, and especially janitor all wrapped up into one, as one former Mr. Mom well remembers.

Since when should such diligence result in corpulence, you have every reason to ask. Since the discovery of electricity, unfortunately.

THE PROBLEM

Our dedication to progress has relegated sweat to the gym. Devote yourself to a career or to maintaining a four-star home front these days, and you can pretty much kiss good old-fashioned exercise good-bye. Automation of the workplace — e-mail, elevators, intercoms, electric pencil sharpeners, and ergonomically perfect office chairs — has made real "work" obsolete. Nor do the calories go up in bonfires as we run our households with food processors, electric mixers, washers and dryers, robotlike vacuum cleaners, and electric knives.

This isn't to suggest that our jobs or family responsibilities are easy, because they most certainly are not. Too often they're downright grueling, in fact — but far more in a mental sense than in a physical one, and therein lies the problem: Exhausted from the shoulders up, we often lack the energy to do much from the shoulders down. Our bodies sit and get fat as our minds get worked to the bone.

THE SOLUTION

So what's anyone with any ambition or feeling of devotion to home sweet home in this new sweat-free world to do? Is it possible to have goals *and* great health? A full plate and fitness, too?

Absolutely, which is the reason for this book. And at the risk of giving away its ending, I'll say right now that the solution is actually quite simple: To make fitness fit in today's push-button society, you're going to have to learn to exercise, as much as anything else, your *imagination*. Your muscle cells and brain cells are going to have to make a pact.

No problem, you say? Muscle-power aside, your brainpower has never been lacking?

To make fitness fit in today's push-button society, you're going to have to learn to exercise . . . your imagination.

Good, because that's what fitness is going to take. And before you stop reading right here and get back to your two-year-old or the *Wall Street Journal*, please know that exercise can be quite enjoyable. Doing your abdominal work while chatting with the members of your car pool, for example, can be far more interesting than doing it at some musty gym. Increasing your cardiovascular endurance on a nature walk with your four-year-old can be far more stimulating than doing it on a walk to nowhere on a treadmill. Firming your fanny while sitting on a straight flush — much more exciting than doing it aboard a stationary bike.

But best of all, this thing called fitness, once you do manage to squeeze it into your jam-packed life, can begin to open your life up, because you'll become more efficient — mentally as well as physically — at everything you do. Can you think of a better way to add more hours to your day than that?

Neither can I, so let's get started by taking a quick look at what this new, more enjoyable journey to higher health is going to involve. Then we'll examine why your fitness efforts may have failed you in the past, followed by a short tour through your body and brain to see what exercise approached the right way can actually do. And finally, before unleashing an arsenal of eminently practical, effective, and even *fun* tips for getting the exercise you need, we'll take a quick diagnostic test to see just how soft our all-too-modern lifestyle has allowed you to become. As demoralizing as the results of that test might be, however, there's good news. Research makes it clear that the people who benefit from exercise *most* are those who've been doing it the *least*. So even if your idea of a workout has been digging the remote out from beneath the pillows of your couch, take heart.

But before we begin to look at *how* to slip in a quick set of muscle-building exercises or stretches, we need to know exactly what exercises to do. Throughout the book, I'll refer you to Appendix A: The Exercises on page 137, where you'll find out just what to do and how to do it correctly. There are more than 50 step-by-step illustrated instructions for simple and effective exercises to work into your day, no matter what it's like and where you spend it. The rest of the book will help you discover *when* you can do them. For your own safety, I strongly recommend that you consult a physician before you begin a new program of physical activity.

The activities recommended in this book are going to have a major impact not just on your shape but also on your chances of living a longer, more productive, and happier life. What's the sense, after all, in allowing yourself to become so short of time that you can't do what it takes to earn more of it? Think about *that* the next time you're asked to put in yet another night of overtime.

The New Fitness
A Kinder, Gentler Approach

Before we get into the nuts and bolts of what it's going to take to retool that overworked but underexercised physique of yours, let's take a moment to examine why the alleged fitness boom has allowed you to fall on such soft times in the first place.

THE HARD FAT TRUTH ABOUT OUR FITNESS HISTORY

First of all, you're by no means alone, if that's any consolation. Despite what all those athletic shoe and low-fat yogurt commercials would have us believe, the fitness boom has actually been a monumental bust. Studies make it embarrassingly clear that we are actually fatter now than we were in the early '60s—back before any of our huffing and puffing in the name of health even began!

Especially hard hit by this inflation, moreover, has been just the age group you'd think would have had the upbringing to avoid it—the baby boomers raised on Ken Cooper's *Aerobics*, Jane Fonda's videos, Jackie Sorensen's calorie-blasting dance steps, and Jack LaLanne's ageless pecs.

**WHILE YOU
READ THIS CHAPTER:**
Contract your abdominals as you
read a paragraph. Release. Repeat at least ten times.

*The rate of obesity among people ages 35 to 45
increased by a whopping 36 percent
between 1962 and 1991.*

These fitness gurus came, but as we now know, they did not conquer. Their message of no pain, no gain backfired, in fact, as shown by numerous surveys, one of the more eye-opening being that of the National Center for Health Statistics (NCHS), reported in 1995. The survey found that as of 1991, the rate of obesity among people ages 35 to 45 had increased by a whopping 36 percent since 1962. (In the early 1960s, as you may recall, only prizefighters jogged, there were no nonfat foods, and cheeseburgers were eaten guilt-free.)

"When substance is separated from hype, the fitness boom was a national obsession that, for most of us, never translated into a way of life," commented *Walking* magazine on the NCHS results.

No kidding. We bought running shoes, stationary bikes, rowing machines, and treadmills in record numbers, but only to make for some extravagant garage sales. Surveys show that of all the people who began to exercise in the '70s and '80s, only 15 percent still maintain their fitness routines today.

So, of course, the big question: Why? If exercise is such an important component of a long and healthy life — and studies continue to show that it most certainly is — why has it fallen so far out of favor?

Failing to Fit Fitness In

Maybe *you* should answer that. Exercise — in the 20- to 30-minute aerobic form we've been told it has to take — is inconvenient, impractical, and time-consuming, is it not? You must change into the proper attire, spend half an hour working up a sweat, then shower and dress again, a total expenditure of several hours, depending on your need for sartorial splendor. And you've got to be in a place that has a locker room or shower.

Nor is exercise much good at helping us get to work on time, pay the bills, keep the house straight, or make dinner for the kids.

No wonder not just you but an estimated 64 percent of us fitness wannabes have chosen to hang up our postworkout towels, according to the President's Council on Physical Fitness and Sports. The pain of fitness we might have been able to handle; it's the *impracticality* and the *monotony* that we could not.

Bored Flabby

Yup, for millions of us, our brains called it quits even before our bodies did. The mindless regimentation inherent in such activities as jogging, stationary cycling, and being strapped to the likes of a rowing machine gave us feelings less of mastery than of slavery. Where was the "empowerment" when empowering activities were no more stimulating than keeping an eagle eye on our heart rates to make sure they didn't drop below a percentage of their precious target zones?

Good question, and one that few exercisers have been able to answer. Surveys of exercise dropouts indicate that if lack of time is exercise-enemy number one, boredom is hot on its heels as number two.

And why not? In a world in which it's hard to find time even to sit down to a meal with the family, sitting down on a stationary bike for an hour at a stretch is a tough pill to swallow, no matter how fantastic the results. We're a nation of doers, raised on the practical wisdom of Ben Franklin and the work ethic of Andrew Carnegie and Horatio Alger. Allotting time each day to pedal, step, or row to nowhere is, was, and maybe always will be an idea more praiseworthy for its intent than its design.

Surveys show that of all the people who began to exercise in the '70s and '80s, only 15 percent still maintain their fitness routines today.

FINALLY: FITNESS REDEFINED!

But enough doom and gloom. The reason we're here is because of the *good* news, which is that there's a new fitness tack in town. Yes, our practicality prayers have been answered, as have our requests for activities more enlightening than watching a digital readout of the minutes crawl by on a stair-climbing machine. The latest word from research labs worldwide is that exercise needn't be such a time-wasting, sweat-producing, brain-numbing affair after all.

Everyday Activities Can Add Up to Fitness

This new understanding started with a landmark study published in the prestigious *Journal of the American Medical Association* back in November 1987. The study found that men who were getting their exercise simply by doing everyday activities, such as walking, gardening, and engaging in light, leisure-time sports, had hearts as healthy as men who were exercising *three* times as much in more traditional ways.

This study, of course, set the stage for numerous others in order to confirm or refute, but the findings have held up. "Moderate levels of activity are as conducive to good health and longevity as more extreme levels," Mr. Aerobics himself, Dr. Ken Cooper, now concedes. Anyone who runs more than 20 miles a week is doing so for reasons other than health, Dr. Cooper says.

Sports medicine specialist Dr. Warren Scott agrees. "We were wrong," says the Stanford University professor and former no-pain, no-gain advocate. "We now know that substantial health benefits can be gained through levels of exercise considerably below what we had once thought. You don't need to be in training for a marathon to maximize your chances of living an optimally long and healthy life."

"Fat cells don't have eyes," says Dr. Bryant Stamford. "They can't see whether you're burning them on a stationary bike or a walk with your dog."

Forget no pain, no gain: Current research shows the path to fitness to be a far kinder and gentler one. The key, simply, is to supplement your normal activity patterns with at least 1,000 calories of additional activity a week (approximately 150 a day). Nearly any activity that requires you to exert yourself beyond a sedentary level will do. For example:

DAY OF THE WEEK	30 MINUTES OF:	CALORIES BURNED*
Monday	Brisk walking	165
Tuesday	Volleyball	170
Wednesday	Ping-Pong (table tennis)	125
Thursday	Bowling	90
Friday	Dancing (disco-style)	170
Saturday	Gardening (weeding and digging)	165
Sunday	Mowing grass (with a push-type rotary mower)	175
		Total: 1,060

*Calorie expenditure given is for a 130-pound person. Figures will be slightly higher for someone weighing more than that, slightly lower for someone weighing less.

Before carting those dumbbells out to the trash once and for all, however, please understand that the new research does not give us license to be comatose. It is quite specific, in fact, about the amount of activity required for good health.

"Between 1,000 and 2,000 calories' worth of activity a week is what the new research is calling for," says Bryant Stamford, Ph.D., director of the Health Promotion and Wellness Center at the University of Louisville. "Some benefits can be accrued from burning as few as 500 calories a week, but for substantial improvement of the cardiovascular system and protection from heart disease, between 1,000 and 2,000 calories appears to be the range to shoot for."

If that sounds like a lot, it's not, because those calories can be burned in virtually *any form* and at *any intensity* you choose, as the chart of activities on page 9 should make abundantly clear.

This is quite a departure from the aerobic doctrine of the '70s and '80s, which, as you may painfully remember, called for workouts that exercised major muscle groups continuously for 20 to 30 minutes at an intensity sufficient to maintain the heart rate within a target zone.

That prescription, as we've seen, is what dug the fitness boom its grave. Finding the *time* to exercise for those 30 sweat-soaked minutes often was harder than the exercise itself.

Go for the Trees, and the Forest Will Come

But that's all perspiration over the dam. We're on a new road to fitness, one that allows for some detours that were not permitted on our fitness trek of old.

"It's now pretty much a case of anything goes," says Dr. Scott. "As long as it's bodily movement, it's exercise, and bits and pieces can add up to being as beneficial as larger and more onerous chunks."

Short Walks Go a Long Way Toward Weight Loss

Interesting proof of the bits-and-pieces approach to fitness was recently presented in a study by researchers from the University of Pittsburgh. When they asked two groups of overweight women to walk for a total of 40 minutes a day — one group continuously, the other in three sessions of however long they wanted — the women who divided their 40 minutes not only made the same cardiovascular advances as the continuously exercising group, but they also lost an average of five pounds *more* over the 20-week period of the study.

The reason?

"In addition to having their shorter walks burn the same number of calories as the longer walks, the women taking the briefer sojourns were less likely to *skip* their walks," the study showed. "The flexibility associated with exercising in short bouts . . . allowed for more consistent exercise participation," concluded the researchers in their 1995 *International Journal of Obesity* report.

That's right, the latest research is showing that we do *not* have to get our exercise all at once, which is maybe the best news of all for the millions of us with schedules as tight as our slacks. Ten minutes here, 10 minutes there — it can all wind up serving the same heart-healthy fat-fighting end.

Consistency. Maybe *that's* the word we should be taping to the refrigerator door instead of this no-pain, no-gain nonsense. Without consistency, exercise is just a drop (of sweat) in a very large bucket. Studies show, for example, that the weekend-warrior syndrome — trying to fit a week's worth of exercise into one day — is as ineffective as it is dangerous. Our bodies prefer to be coaxed rather than coerced. And while some research does suggest that higher activity levels may bestow additional gains, exercise physiologist Bryant Stamford says, "The gains are very small, and probably not worth the average person's pursuit considering the time, effort, and vastly increased risks of injury they entail."

So accessible are the rewards of moderate exercise, in fact, that two doctors reporting several years ago in the no-nonsense *New England Journal of Medicine* determined that the average person could enjoy virtually all the same life-extending benefits as even a die-hard fitness buff by

66 There's no way I can carve an hour out of my day for exercising. But I do try to make the most out of every movement I make. When I take a load of laundry downstairs, I go up and down an extra time before I go upstairs for good. When I bend over to pick up toys, I make it into a stretching workout by touching my toes and holding it for a few seconds. As a result, I feel much more enthusiastic about those chores, and all those little bits of exercise really do make a difference. 99

SANDRA, mother of four

*Virtually all the life-extending benefits of exercise
can be enjoyed simply by climbing stairs
for six minutes a day.*

— are you ready for this? — simply climbing stairs for six minutes a day.

Taking their calculations one step further, the doctors estimated that four additional seconds of life stand to be gained for every stair climbed.

With those figures in mind, we should learn to disdain elevators and escalators. And maybe cabs, subways, cross-town buses, riding lawn mowers, and golf carts, too. Life-extending exercise is so much more available to us than the amenities of our all-too civilized lives would lead us to believe. As the American Council on Exercise says of stair-climbing, "Your building may have a health club you don't even know about."

So take heart and read on. A more leisurely road to fitness is out there, as even the U.S. government's Office of the Surgeon General now agrees. In a statement made as recently as the summer of 1996, the amount of exercise called for was an eminently doable 150 calories' worth a day—the equivalent of a leisurely 30-minute walk or any of the other highly user-friendly activities listed in the chart on page 9. The road to fitness, you see, needn't be so steep and narrow after all.

EXERCISE UNDER THE MICROSCOPE: HEAD-TO-TOE HEALTH BENEFITS

Okay, so maybe exercise doesn't have to be such a pain in the gluteus maximus after all. But besides putting a nice flush on your face and burning some calories, what can it actually *do?* Is it really the "magic bullet" that some doctors, dressed in their name-brand running shoes and shorts, seem so eager for us to believe?

Yes and no. Yes, exercise is a "bullet" when it comes to combating obesity and shooting down risks of most major diseases, but it's by no means a magic one. Exercise works its "miracles" 100 percent naturally, by enabling the body and the mind to function as fully as they were intended.

The benefits of exercise have been known for thousands of years, long before people like Richard Simmons and some savvy sneaker companies started singing its praises. "A man falls into ill health as a result of not caring to exercise," wrote the Greek philosopher Aristotle some 300 years before the birth of Christ, an opinion echoed by notable healers ever since.

Exercise and the Body: Your Cells Are Dying for It

Our bodies, for an estimated 500 million years, got exercise virtually all day long, because our very lives depended on it. A consequence of *not* keeping constantly on the go, in fact, might have been no supper, or perhaps *becoming* supper. Only very recently — since the industrial advances at the beginning of this century — have our bodies had to deal with the strange new stresses of sedentary life. That's a lot of biological momentum with nowhere to go.

Our bodies have evolved into their present forms *because* of exercise, after all; why should we think they can suddenly do without it?

Not Exercising Is Hazardous to Your Health

Adequate physical activity has been found to be so important to good health that a recent report in the *Archives of Internal Medicine* warned that insufficient levels of exercise should be considered as detrimental to health as — believe it or not — smoking half a pack of cigarettes a day.

To add to the alarming findings of that report, doctors presented statistics a year later in the *Journal of the American Medical Association* showing that people who don't exercise, when compared to those who exercise moderately, could expect their risk of dying prematurely to double.

Exercise is more critical for basic survival, both physical and mental, than some of us wedded to our La-Z-Boys would ever have suspected, and a quick look at what it actually does on a cellular level should explain why. Only 30 minutes of moderate physical activity each day are needed to help unleash the cellular angst brought on by inactivity. Bear that in mind as you review the following summary of exercise's proven benefits:

1. Exercise increases circulation by widening blood vessels and even creating new ones, thus reducing risks of heart attack and stroke. In addition, it boosts physical and mental stamina by improving the delivery of oxygen and other vital nutrients to virtually every cell in the body — those of the brain included.

2. Exercise lowers blood pressure, a major risk factor for heart attack, aneurysms, glaucoma, and stroke.

3. Exercise improves the ratio of good (HDL) to bad (LDL) cholesterol in the blood, thus reducing the risk of heart attack due to arterial blockage caused by the accumulation of plaque on artery walls.

4. Exercise helps the body make better use of insulin, thus substantially reducing the risk of type II (adult-onset) diabetes.

5. Exercise improves lung function and hence physical as well as mental stamina by increasing the amount of oxygen in the blood.

6. Exercise helps bolster the immune system, thus increasing protection against everything from cancer to the common cold.

7. Exercise strengthens bones by boosting their uptake of calcium, thus dramatically reducing the risk of osteoporosis (a major problem for women following menopause).

8. Exercise helps keep joints healthy, thus reducing the risk of osteoarthritis.

Take a look at the 19 reasons listed in the box that starts above. If it took the last item to get your interest, so be it. The point is that the benefits of exercise are so extensive that there's something in it for everybody. Whether you're a homemaker just wanting more energy (and maybe more patience with the kids), a would-be VIP wanting more pep to climb a

9. Exercise helps strengthen the muscles of the lower back, thus reducing the risk of chronic back pain.

10. Exercise tones and strengthens muscles of the arms, legs, and abdomen, thus improving endurance as well as appearance.

11. Exercise speeds reaction time, reducing risks of driving mishaps as well as accidents around the home.

12. Exercise improves coordination, lowering the risks associated with falling (especially among the elderly).

13. Exercise aids digestion and hence optimal absorption of vital nutrients.

14. Exercise helps promote intestinal regularity, thus reducing the risk of cancers of the colon.

15. Exercise helps burn body fat and maintain healthy weight, thus boosting energy levels and improving appearance as well as reducing risks of diabetes, high blood pressure, harmful wear and tear on joints, and even certain types of cancer (i.e., breast cancer in women and prostate cancer in men).

16. Exercise aids restful, higher-quality sleep.

17. Exercise lowers the resting heart rate by increasing the amount of blood pumped by each of the heart's contractions, thus saving the heart as many as 50,000 beats a day, and 17 million in a year!

18. Exercise helps slow the aging process by improving blood circulation and hence the delivery of vital nutrients *to*, and the removal of metabolic waste *from*, virtually every cell in the body — skin included!

19. Exercise improves sexual performance by boosting physical endurance and flexibility as well as body image and self-esteem.

corporate ladder, or a senior citizen looking for the energy to enjoy retirement, exercise is your answer.

No matter what condition your body is in, beginning to exercise right now will improve your health and the quality of your life — because you'll feel better, mentally as well as physically.

Exercise and the Brain: Neurons Like the Sweat, Too

Exercise does more than give our bodies their biological due; it also benefits our brains, because our brains depend on our bodies for their most vital needs. Regular exercise helps keep the brain better fed by giving it a steadier flow of glucose — the same stuff that fuels muscles — plus freer flows of oxygen by helping to maintain cleaner blood vessels. The result is not just greater mental endurance, some studies indicate, but also enhanced creativity and intelligence.

So effective can exercise be at pumping up the brain that even the bottom-line business sector is beginning to realize its potential. As Robert K. Cooper, author of *The Performance Edge*, says, "An active lifestyle is a cornerstone not just of good health but also of highly productive work. People who make a point of fitting an adequate amount of physical activity in their lives not only get more done in less time, they're better at handling stress and they tend to be more imaginative when it comes to solving work-related problems."

Exercise is showing itself to be such an effective performance-enhancer in today's corporate jungle, in fact, that it's getting recommended right up there with the pinstriped suit as a requirement for getting ahead. "After working with thousands of people, I now recommend a regular exercise program as the single best way both to facilitate creativity and increase resistance to stress," reports UCLA professor of medicine Thomas E. Backer, M.D., in *Health and Fitness in the Workplace*.

Then, too, there's the all-important stress-fighting component of exercise for an even further mental edge, Dr. Cooper says. He cites studies showing that regular physical exercise can be a powerful antidote to stress by burning off tension-induced chemicals before they can do their mind-frying and artery-clogging damage. Exercise does this by using these stress-induced chemicals as *fuel* — a case of waste management par excellence.

By getting the body to run better, exercise improves the functioning of the mind. The brain may think it's the boss, but without a healthy body supporting it, it's about as powerful as a candidate with no votes. Research now concludes that regular physical exercise can improve brain function by:

- **Improving memory.** Memory depends on good communication among all parts of the brain, and exercise appears to help keep the wires (blood vessels) responsible for that communication in good condition.

- **Increasing problem-solving ability and creativity.** The brain cell benefiting from exercise may also be the more clever brain cell, as attested by recent research with business executives — plus the cerebral track records of such avid exercisers as Wordsworth, Thoreau, Einstein, and Aristotle.

- **Creating stronger immunity to stress.** "Exercise appears to burn up excess stress chemicals by using them for energy expressed outwardly rather than inwardly, where they can do harm," explains cardiologist Robert S. Elliot.

- **Helping us to keep our chins up.** And not just over the bar. Exercise is a potent mood-elevator, as shown in clinical studies with depressed mental patients. To be thanked: the 100 percent all-natural uppers called endorphins.

- **Improving stamina.** Let's face it: It's tough to be smart when you're pooped. Exercise can give the physical boost that intellectual stamina cannot do without.

*Exercise can be like push-ups
for the brain.*

Regular exercise can also help elevate the spirits and nour-ish self-esteem by keeping the blood infused with the body's natural mood-boosters, called endorphins. By a similar mecha-nism, it can often help prevent and even alleviate depression.

New research is showing that exercise may even—and here's a benefit none of us can afford to forget—help enhance our *memories*, especially as we age. As much as our memories are made of good times and bad, you see, they need an adequate blood flow within the brain, which exercise ensures with every step we take.

So now that you know all of its benefits, are you ready to learn what fitness is actually going to require?

Good, because you're likely to be pleasantly surprised.

The New Approach to Fitness

The sales pitch is over, because it's my hope that by now you've bought it. What still needs to be addressed, however, are recommendations for how and when to fit this potentially unwieldy thing called exercise into your already hectic life. It does continue to trip up millions of us daily, don't forget, so we must be doing something wrong.

For an exercise program to succeed in becoming a permanent and worthwhile endeavor, it's going to have to do two things:

1. It's going to have to fit comfortably into your life.
2. It's going to have to work.

A do-or-die approach to exercise is as doomed to fail as even the most diligent use of something electronic to shrink the thighs. So often fitness programs don't last because we undertake them aiming for a Mercedes, and lose interest when it becomes clear that all we may have time for is a Honda.

To which we say: A Honda beats whatever heap is currently transporting your bones around. Research continues to come in even as this book is going to print showing that even

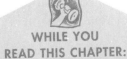

**WHILE YOU
READ THIS CHAPTER:**
Contract your stomach muscles and curl your buttocks forward for a pelvic tilt. Hold and release. Repeat five times.

a little exercise, so long as it's done consistently, can be significantly better than no exercise at all. That's basically all the motivation you should need. The rest — actually fitting that exercise into your life — is going to be up to you.

THE MOST IMPORTANT FITNESS INGREDIENT OF ALL: IMAGINATION

If there's one key ingredient that's been lacking in the ways exercise has been sold in years past, it has been permission to exercise the imagination. There's been an abundance of encouragement and instruction to exercise our biceps, triceps, and abs, that's for sure, but too often it has been given within guidelines that are restrictive to the point of being prohibitive. Do we really need a 2,000-pound weight machine to work our pecs, or something available for three "easy" payments to tighten our tummies?

Of course not. It's the movement that counts, not the machinery, and there are far more ways to get that movement than would be economically wise for manufacturers of exercise devices to admit.

The same holds true for the *time* normally recommended for exercise, and for the attire. Exercise for at least 30 continuous minutes within a target heart rate, we're told. Wear Lycra because it breathes.

Baloney. As long as *you're* breathing, that's what matters. It's time we stopped making exercise so needlessly and extravagantly complicated.

A Whole Greater Than the Sum of Its Parts

As you may recall from the first chapter, a study done with overweight women by researchers from the University of Pittsburgh found that women permitted to divide their exercise time into 10-minute increments lost more weight than women instructed to exercise continuously 40 minutes at a time. It was a very important and highly suggestive finding, but not just because of its implications on a biochemical level regarding the burning of fat: The women who lost more weight did so because their shorter exercise segments permitted them to exercise something more than their quadriceps: They were allowed the flexibility to exercise their imaginations.

Shorter periods of exercise can be easier to fit into your day than a long workout. Inadvertently, the study had discovered something vitally important yet long overlooked regarding exercise compliance in this madcap world we live in — namely, that as important as *what* we need to do for fitness is *how* we're permitted to do it. The women assigned to the shorter exercise periods were found to be far more creative than the other group at fitting their exercise into their daily routines. "The flexibility associated with exercising in short segments may allow for more consistent exercise participation," observed the researchers in their *International Journal of Obesity* report.

If you can relate to this discovery, you're in good company. Exercise programs of the past have *not* encouraged us to be creative, but rather have wanted us to follow robotically in the steps of any number of glistening exercise gurus.

You probably have some stories of your own to corroborate the drawbacks of this all-too-military approach to fitness, but maybe you'll relate to this experience I'd like to tell you about. It pertains to a woman named Martha, a 36-year-old working mother of two whose initial failures followed by success document the advantages of approaching exercise creatively.

Martha, by her own admission, had become a diet junkie. She would latch on to a weight-loss plan, any weight-loss plan, with the fervor of an addict, only to fail when it became clear that what she was attempting simply was not biologically possible, much less safe.

But then Martha began to hear of the miracles of exercise for losing weight, and she went at that like a house afire as well. She hired a cleaning service and a baby-sitter, and joined a state-of-the-art health club with the intention of working out for at least an hour a day, five days a week.

Well, she joined the health club, but nothing went according to plan. At first she was intimidated, and didn't enjoy how she stacked up against so many women built like Barbie. Next, she became bored by the workouts, in addition to discovering that watching the oscillation of her excess flesh in a full-length mirror was not one of the more uplifting experiences in life.

Finally, Martha was in fact *injured* by her health-club effort when she dropped a 40-pound dumbbell on her foot, ending her fitness quest on a sour note indeed.

She didn't shed pounds or inches, regrettably, but she did lose plenty of dollars — about 900 of them, what with the membership fee and the costs of the cleaning service and the baby-sitter, who had a major appetite for the more costly contents of Martha's refrigerator.

This is not meant to disparage health clubs, don't get me wrong. For people who have the time and the personality for them, supervised fitness programs can be wonderful. But for people who prefer more autonomy, or who have family responsibilities, or who don't feel they're at their best in skimpy outfits, clubs may call for more effort than fitness requires.

But let's get back to Martha, because her story's far from over. Her failure helped her find success. "I guess out of necessi-

According to a survey by American Sports Data, only one out of every three individuals who join a health club work out 100 days or more a year.

ty as much as anything else," she says, "I started looking for ways to incorporate some of the exercises I had learned at the health club into my everyday life. I started using the basement stairs for a five-minute cardiovascular workout before taking my shower in the morning. Then I added some exercises for my arms that I do on the steering wheel of my car at traffic lights on the way to work. At lunch I started adding a short walk, which also helped me limit the amount I ate, and at night I started doing stretching exercises on the floor while watching TV with the kids."

Nice job, Martha! Martha rescued herself with her imagination. She came up with a workout on the fly that was covering the same essential bases as her health-club ordeal. Yes, she was taking the whole day, in a sense, to do it, but she was fitting it in, and it was working!

"And it doesn't cost me a cent," says Martha, who is now 10 pounds lighter. "The stretching that I do with my kids at night is one of the high points of my day, in fact. They love to do the stretches along with me, and when we're done we reward ourselves with a healthy, low-fat treat."

Are You Too Busy to Breathe?

If Martha's fitness solution appears too easy to be true, it's only because you've been looking at fitness through eyes perhaps blurred by the sweat you've thought it must produce. Or maybe you've put it off because of the unaffordable blocks of time you've been taught it must demand. Please *forget* those constraints if they've been holding you back from being more active. The latest research leaves no doubt that fitness can be attained in a wider variety of forms, at lesser intensities, and for shorter periods of time than formerly believed.

As sports medicine specialist Warren Scott, M.D., of Stanford University puts it, "We now know that the benefits of physical activity can be cumulative, that anything is better than nothing, and that activities done separately from one another definitely can add up even though they might not in and of themselves meet the durations of 20 to 30 minutes once prescribed.

"This should come as great news for people who in the past might have been avoiding exercise for being unable to find what they thought were the needed amounts of time," Dr. Scott says. "We can now say to those people that they're too busy to exercise only if they're, well, too busy to breathe."

THE THREE BASIC COMPONENTS OF FITNESS: NOTHING TO SWEAT OVER

Martha's collection of makeshift maneuvers worked for her because it included each of the three components that a well-balanced fitness program requires:

 1. *Cardiovascular or aerobic component* — for improving function of the heart and lungs, burning calories, and helping to control cholesterol levels, blood pressure, and stress

 2. *Strength-building component* — for maintaining good muscular firmness and shape

 3. *Flexibility component* — for greater mobility along with relief from stiffness and stress

These are the raw ingredients of fitness, to be cooked up in any way you find most palatable to your particular responsibilities and lifestyle. Bits and pieces of each type of activity, like pennies in a piggy bank, can add up; they count just as much as the same amount of time spent at these activities all at once.

You're too busy to exercise only if you're too busy to breathe.

Ingredient #1: Cardiovascular/Aerobic Exercise

Yes, this is the type of exercise that started the fitness movement off and running, and it includes, quite simply, activities continuous and rhythmic in nature that work major muscle groups (such as the arms and/or the legs) sufficiently to strengthen the respiratory system and heart. Exercise of this type — partly because it can be done for extended periods but also because it helps the body develop fat-burning enzymes — is generally regarded as the best for controlling weight. Because of its continual employment of the circulatory system, aerobic exercise also is considered the best type for lowering blood pressure, reducing serum cholesterol and triglycerides, and helping to alleviate and build resistance to stress — all significant factors in reducing the risk of heart attack and stroke.

Do we need to run races or chain ourselves to a ski machine for hours to reap the benefits? No. All we need is a total of about 30 minutes a day, divided into whatever time quantities we like. Best of all, this potent health-enhancer can be found *nearly everywhere.*

Or at least it *could* be, "if we'd just approach more of our everyday activities with a little more oomph," says exercise physiologist Bryant Stamford. "So many of our everyday activities have the potential for being far greater forms of exercise than we let them. By increasing the intensity with which we approach many of our household chores and leisure time activities only slightly, we could increase the health benefits they produce quite substantially."

Activities that otherwise would be good merely for being mild calorie-burners could become officially aerobic, in other words. They would be strenuous enough to raise the heart rate and oxygen consumption to levels capable of measurably improving not just our fitness but also our odds against most major diseases.

"This isn't to suggest that there aren't significant benefits to virtually any physical activity we undertake, even if it's just

Your target heart rate is the range of your maximum heart rate in which your body is burning oxygen and your heart is being strengthened. To determine your target heart rate, first use the following formula to find your approximate maximum rate:

220 - Age = Maximum Heart Rate (MHR)

164

Plug your MHR into the next formulas to learn your target heart rate range. Most exercise programs stipulate that to reach and maintain cardiovascular fitness, you should work out at only 60 to 85 percent of your maximum heart rate.

MHR x .60 = Lower limit of target heart rate range — *98.40*
MHR x .85 = Upper limit of target heart rate range — *139.40*

Stay within this range to maximize the fat-burning benefits of aerobic exercise.

---

washing the dishes," Dr. Stamford says. "There is, however, a threshold beyond which health benefits appear to increase rather dramatically."

That threshold is the target heart rate you may have heard mentioned in connection with some of your fitness efforts of old. Put simply, it's a level of exertion capable of producing measurable improvements in the cardiovascular system — an increase in the amount of blood the heart is able to pump with each stroke and a decrease in your pulse rate while at rest. Calorie-burning also increases proportionally to the amount of passion with which we approach any given activity, so it's not just our hearts that benefit when we pick up the pace — our figures do, too.

But for a go-getter like you, that shouldn't be a problem, right? The fact that you're so busy needn't hinder your fitness: It can *help* by motivating you to employ the levels of exertion that promote fitness best!

The Components of Fitness: Easy as 1, 2, 3

Talk to any experienced camper, and you'll learn that it takes three logs to make a good fire. Well, three is an important number in fitness, too. A well-rounded fitness program should include the following three components. It doesn't matter how you fit exercise into your busy life so long as you do activities that benefit you in these three ways.

EXERCISE CATEGORY	BENEFITS	EXAMPLES
Cardiovascular/ Aerobic Exercise	Improves function of heart and lungs. Burns calories and fat. Helps to control cholesterol levels and blood pressure. Relieves stress. Improves efficiency and endurance.	Walking, running, swimming, bicycling, climbing stairs, dancing, hiking, sports, raking leaves, mowing grass
Strengthening Exercise	Shapes and tones muscles. Helps you burn calories while at rest. Strengthens bones, reducing risk of osteoporosis.	Lifting weights, push-ups, pull-ups, isometric exercises, sit-ups, leg lifts
Flexibility Exercise	Greater mobility. Provides relief from stiffness and stress. Keeps muscles loose, reducing risk of injury. Affords relief from aches and pains related to aging.	Yoga, dance movements, all stretching exercises (see Appendix A), reaching, bending

Ingredient #2: Strength-Building Exercise

There's more to fitness than just a healthy heart, of course. You need some muscle power to go with it, and not just for moving refrigerators or carrying heavy bags of groceries. Muscle is vitally important for weight control, because muscle is the best calorie-burning tissue the body has. It's more effective than fat even when at rest, and its calorie-burning ability can leap as much as 20-fold when called into action. The more muscle we have, therefore, the better at burning calories we're going to be — even while just watching the evening news!

This is why people who do only aerobic exercise, which is not effective at building muscle, tend to gain weight so quickly if they stop: With relatively little muscle mass to fall back on, their calorie-burning is dependent almost entirely on what they use up during their aerobic workouts. If they're suddenly derailed by an injury — or an exceptionally busy schedule — boom: Calorie-burning stops and fat production begins if appropriate dietary cutbacks are not made.

Maybe crawling inside a muscle to see what it really looks like will help illustrate why this is so.

Muscle tissue is composed of two types of fibers. Within each of the 650 muscles we have, two types of muscle fibers lie side by side: fast-twitch and slow-twitch. When a muscle is exercised aerobically (that is, in the continuous, rhythmic fashion mentioned above), it is primarily the muscle's slow-twitch fibers that get called into action. These fibers gain in endurance from such activity, but they do *not* increase appreciably in strength or size — thus, the birdlike physiques of most good marathoners. Despite their grueling 100-plus-mile-a-week training regimens, there is no appreciable increase in the muscular bulk of their legs. Their legs often get even thinner, in fact, as unused *fast-twitch* fibers shrink and in some cases even die.

When a muscle is exercised in a strength-building way, however, fast-twitch fibers get the call, and their response is to increase in size. This is why the folks in those muscle-building magazines look the way they do. Their exercise routines focus primarily on the development of their muscles' fast-twitch fibers, and yes, some amazing growth can be the result.

Muscle tissue
burns more calories than
fat tissue, even when your body is at rest.

But hold the dumbbells — who wants that Arnold Schwarzenegger look, especially if you're a woman who just wants to be slimmer?

Be careful. Studies show that the losses in muscle mass and strength that we suffer with age are due almost entirely to atrophy of our fast-twitch, not our slow-twitch, fibers. This is because our slow-twitchers get called upon by even the most minimal exertions. Our fast-twitch fibers, by contrast, sit around and do little more than twiddle their thumbs as we age, eventually disappearing entirely if we don't remind them we know they're there. This disappearing act can begin in earnest as early as our 30s, and if left unchecked can progress to truly a pathetic degree. Surveys show, for example, that over one-quarter of American men and *two-thirds* of American women cannot lift more than 10 pounds by the time they reach age 75. Fast-twitch neglect has been targeted as the primary cause.

Some loss of muscle and strength with age is inevitable, don't get me wrong. But when someone like fitness dynamo Jack LaLanne can commemorate his 65th birthday by swimming 1½ miles towing 65 rowboats loaded with 65,000 pounds of wood pulp — while wearing handcuffs! — it's clear that

Slow-Twitch and Fast-Twitch Muscle Builders

Aerobic activity develops slow-twitch muscle fiber, which improves endurance. Strengthening movements develop fast-twitch muscle fibers, which can ultimately disappear if not used. Many activities exercise both.

SLOW-TWITCH ACTIVITY	FAST-TWITCH ACTIVITY
Running for a bus	Lifting groceries
Walking the dog	Carrying laundry
Swimming with kids	Lifting a small child
Dancing	Shoveling snow
Playing basketball	Isometric exercises
Rowing a boat	Rowing a boat
Climbing stairs	Climbing stairs
Riding a bicycle	Riding a bicycle

many of us are letting Father Time get away with far more than we have to.

Don't worry, though. I'm not going to be recommending the daily diet of push-ups that have earned ageless Jack his legendary acclaim. I'll simply be showing you how to incorporate the recommended 5 to 10 minutes of strength-building activities naturally — even advantageously — into your harried life.

Ingredient #3: Flexibility Exercise

Flexibility, as it applies to physical fitness, is defined as the ability to use a part of the body through its full range of motion. This does not mean that we need to be as limber as a contortionist, however. It simply means that we need to keep our muscles and joints mobile enough to avoid discomforts that — especially for those of us with jobs that have us sitting all day — can leave us feeling about as limber as the Tin Man. Muscles and connective tissue (ligaments and tendons) tend to shorten and tighten with age even in the habitually active, so you can imagine the liabilities for those of us who are desk-bound. Chronic back pain, neck pain, shoulder pain, headaches, bad posture, undue fatigue, and heightened vulnerability to stress all can result from muscles and joints simply too uptight for their own good.

Fortunately, many of the exercises and activities I'll be recommending for building cardiovascular endurance and muscular strength can in themselves help keep you loose, but it's important also to have an arsenal of stretches for particular problems caused by sedentary endeavors — things such as that why-do-I-suddenly-feel-like-I'm-made-of-concrete sensation that comes over you after one too many hours glued to a computer screen. Or that feeling of not being able to touch

Staying flexible helps to prevent back, neck, and shoulder pain, as well as headaches and fatigue.

your knees much less your toes after two butt-paralyzing hours spent in the bleachers watching Susie's extra-inning softball game.

HOW FIT OR UNFIT ARE YOU?

But before doing exercise of any sort, we have some diagnostic work to do. We need to find out just what sort of physical condition you're in, because if you're rock-solid already — finding time to exercise strenuously for at least 30 minutes, three or more times a week — maybe you don't need this book. Perhaps you can stop reading right here, pass these pages on to someone who does need them, and head off to the health club or home gym for your next workout. I'm happy for you if that's the case.

But chances are that's not how it is. You might be one of the estimated 64 percent of Americans who don't get the amount of physical activity that studies show can significantly improve health and extend life. Maybe your life is an average and yet ominously automated one, complete with electric garage-door opener, sit-down lawnmower, TV remote, and even an electric toothbrush. And, of course, maybe you consider yourself too busy to do much about it.

If that's the case, then this book most definitely *is* for you, but we need to find out. So what do you say we take an analytical look at the amount of physical activity in your average day.

Yes, I could be asking you to do push-ups, a shuttle run, and as many sit-ups as you can in 60 seconds to measure your fitness, but tests like that too often miss the point. You could do well on such a test thanks to good genes alone, yet still be leading a life of debauchery destined for the cardiac-care unit at any time. Research makes it very clear, in fact, that it's the activity we get, more so than the athletic ability we've been given or past glories we have enjoyed, that has the greater impact on our health.

You're as fit as you are active, and by measuring what you do on an average day, you can reliably gauge your level of fitness. Ready? Then good luck and no cheating, please. Record the point value for each answer as shown. If a question doesn't apply to you, go on to the next without adding anything to your score.

1. On an average day, I climb and descend an average of about ____ flights of stairs. (Consider a flight to be 12 steps.)
   a.) 1–5 (1 point)
   b.) 6–10 (2 points)
   c.) more than 10 (4 points)

2. I have a desk job but leave my desk regularly to run errands, greet visitors, attend meetings, etc., at least ____ times an hour on an average day.
   a.) 6 times or fewer per hour (0 points)
   b.) more than 6 times per hour (1 point)

3. My job requires that I be on my feet *and moving* an average of about ____ hours a day.
   a.) 1–2 hours (2 points)
   b.) 2–3 hours (3 points)
   c.) 3–4 hours (4 points)
   d.) 4 or more hours (6 points)

4. My job requires that I be on my feet basically *standing* for approximately ____ hours a day.
   a.) less than 4 hours (0 points)
   b.) 4–6 hours (1 point)
   c.) 6–8 hours (2 points)
   d.) 8 or more hours (3 points)

5. On an average day, I walk about ____ miles, either recreationally or as part of my job.
   a.) 1–2 miles (2 points)
   b.) 2–3 miles (4 points)
   c.) 3–4 miles (6 points)
   d.) 4 or more miles (10 points)

6. I spend about ____ hours a week tending a garden or lawn or doing home improvements such as carpentry and

painting. (Points assume year-round activity; if seasonal, cut points in half.)
  a.) 1–2 hours (1 point)
  b.) 2–3 hours (2 points)
  c.) 3–4 hours (3 points)
  d.) 4–5 hours (4 points)
  e.) 5 or more hours (5 points)

7. I am a parent who assumes primary responsibility for a preschool child. (Add 50 percent of points for each additional child.)
  a.) Child and parent at home all day (5 points)
  b.) Child spends half day in day-care center (3 points)
  c.) Child spends full day in day-care center (1 point)

8. My job is physically demanding (lifting, carrying, shoveling, climbing) for _____ hours a day. (Don't count time spent while shooting the breeze, please.)
  a.) 1–2 hours (3 points)
  b.) 2–3 hours (5 points)
  c.) 3–4 hours (7 points)
  d.) 4–5 hours (9 points)
  e.) 5 or more hours (12 points)

9. I engage in sporting activities such as tennis, softball, basketball, or (cartless) golf, or I go dancing an average of about _____ hours a week. (Year-round activity is assumed, even though the sports may change. If the activity is seasonal, divide the points earned accordingly.)
  a.) 1–2 hours (1 point)
  b.) 2–3 hours (2 points)
  c.) 3–4 hours (3 points)
  d.) 4 or more hours (5 points)

10. I do household chores (laundry, cleaning, cooking) an average of _____ hours a week.
  a.) 1–2 hours (1 point)
  b.) 2–3 hours (2 points)
  c.) 3–4 hours (3 points)
  d.) 4–5 hours (4 points)
  e.) 5 or more hours (6 points)

Scoring: Add up your points and match with the corresponding description.

11+: Commendable. Even though you are not engaged in a formal exercise program, chances are good that you are getting an adequate amount of physical activity in your average day. This does not mean that more activity would not be better, however, especially if you're trying to control your weight, so pay attention to the advice that lies ahead.

5 to 10 points: Not commendable. You're on the edge — not a couch potato, but too close for comfort. Building more activity into your day will improve your health, give you more energy, help you lose body fat, and help you relax.

0 to 4 points: Reprehensible. You're over the edge, a couch potato all-star, and your health could be suffering accordingly. Please pay close attention to what lies ahead, as your life, quite literally, could depend on it.

(Thanks to Dr. Bryant Stamford, Director of the Health Promotion and Wellness Center at the University of Louisville, for his help in creating this test.)

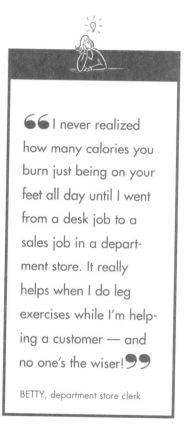

❝I never realized how many calories you burn just being on your feet all day until I went from a desk job to a sales job in a department store. It really helps when I do leg exercises while I'm helping a customer — and no one's the wiser!❞

BETTY, department store clerk

Making Fitness Fit
Morning

T ime for a quick summary, because just a few short paragraphs from now it's going to be time to put all this stuff to work.

We've seen that a balanced fitness program requires three basic elements:

 A cardiovascular or aerobic component for weight control and the health of the circulatory system.

 A strength component for maintaining muscle mass and thus an active weight-controlling metabolism.

 Flexibility maneuvers for keeping limber and pain-free enough to want to be active in the first place.

And yes, I know. Despite all we've been saying about how easy it can be, you're still not convinced that you're going to be able to find the time. How, simply by using your imagination, are you going to lengthen your day by the 30 minutes these fitness endeavors require?

**WHILE YOU
READ THIS CHAPTER:**
Take a stair-climbing break.
Climb up and down a 12-step flight. Repeat at least 3 times.

I'll tell you how. You're going to do as all great running backs in the game of football do: You're going to learn to look for openings. Any openings. Five minutes here. Ten minutes there. It can all *add up* regardless of intensity or duration, remember, because the new research shows that we can get our fitness in "nibbles" rather than just those long and hard-to-swallow "feasts" of old.

So relax, pay attention, and feel free to come up with some ideas of your own. Your goal each day should be to "consume" at least 20 minutes of cardiovascular activity, 5 to 10 minutes of strength-building, and 5 to 10 minutes of stretching. That might sound like a lot, but it needn't *feel* like a lot if you can just learn to do *what* you can *when* you can. The only limit to what you can achieve with this system is — as I've said before — your imagination.

Doing aerobic activity usually means that you can't do any other activity at the same time. That's one reason many of us don't do it more often. But strength and flexibility exercises can be squeezed in while you're doing other things, and that's where your imagination must be especially active.

So let's get creative, and let's start with your most frenetic time of all: the morning, when, if you're like most hard-working Americans, you barely have time to butter your toast. In chapters 4

> **❝** I do stretches before I get out of bed, then I roll onto the floor for some stomach crunches and push-ups before I get dressed. After that I do a quick workout on the rowing machine, or if it's summertime, I go for a swim in the lake. I'm a real bear if I miss my morning routine for more than a day. **❞**
>
> GLENN, junior high school teacher

and 5, we'll look at how to squeeze similar fit-bits into your noon and evening hours, but for now let's start with the morning. If you can squeeze fitness into this time, the rest should be easy.

We all have different feelings about the morning: Some of us love it, others of us just do what we can to get through it. Therefore, I'm offering many alternatives for your morning workout.

But even if you're about as much of a morning person as Dracula, take heart: You can mix and match your exercise alternatives to create an approach that suits you and that fits into your schedule. No exercise program works if you don't do it, so choosing an activity that you really enjoy and that conforms to your time limitations is very important. Do you cringe at the first glimpse of sunlight when you fetch the morning paper from the front stoop? Then by all means pick indoor exercises that get your blood circulating before you open that door. Are you energized by the smell of fresh air? Then get outside right away and walk, jog, run, bike, or skate before your shower. Whatever it is that gets your motor running, *do it* — and it will jump-start you for the day ahead.

FLEXIBILITY EXERCISES FOR THE A.M.

As we've conceded, many of us find ourselves nearly comatose upon arising. If that's you, some nice and easy stretches will help get you going painlessly, even pleasantly. In addition, they can help prime you for whatever tedious tasks your day may have in store.

Stretches can be worked into your mornings without changing your routine at all. Most can even be done before you get out of bed. Get into the habit of doing the same stretches everyday upon awakening, and they will become just that: a habit that you do without having to think

Even before getting out of bed you can polish off some if not all of your flexibility requirement for the day. You'll also get your blood circulating to help get you on your way.

- **The Jackknife.** Lying on your back, bend one leg at the knee, foot on the bed. Grasp behind the knee of the bent leg and pull it as close as possible into your chest, keeping your other leg in full contact with the bed if you can. Hold the tucked position for 20 seconds, then switch to the other knee. Repeat the sequence five times. This stretch is particularly good for loosening the muscles of the lower back, which can be especially stiff in the morning if you suffer from low back pain due to arthritis. (See Appendix A for illustration.)

- **The Long Stretch.** Lie on your back with your arms at your sides, thumbs up. Tilt your pelvis until your lower back is pressed into the bed; hold. Press your heels out and slowly raise your arms over your head to the point of comfort. Continue to breathe as you hold this position for 30 seconds. Then relax the legs, and keeping your pelvis tilted, return your arms to the starting position.

- **The Trunk Stretch.** This stretch helps to increase flexibility in the upper body. Get on your hands and knees. Keeping your arms straight in front of you, slowly sit back onto your heels while pressing down with your palms. (Your head should end up lowered between your arms.) Hold for 30 seconds, breathing normally. (Tuck your pillow behind your knee crease if this feels tight.)

---

about it. The same is true of the shower, a place that is especially well suited for stretching since the hot water helps loosen muscles even more.

Be sure to do stretches slowly and without bouncing to avoid the risk of muscular and/or connective tissue damage. Never stretch to the point of feeling pain. Finally, remember to breathe as you stretch.

Stretching in the Bathroom

Many people find stretching in the shower more comfortable because of the moist heat, which soothes and relaxes stiff muscles. Here are some other ideas for getting the most out of your bathroom time.

- While brushing your teeth, slowly rotate your upper body at the hips as far in each direction as you can. Good for loosening the muscles of the lower back and hips.

- While in the shower, stretch the muscles of your neck, shoulders, and upper back by gently tilting your head as far as you can to one side, then forward, and then to the other side. Repeat several times.

- Shoulder Rotations feel especially good under hot water. (See Appendix A.)

- When out of the shower, touch your toes (or at least get as close as you can) as you're toweling off. Keep your legs straight and be careful not to bounce. Good for stretching the hamstrings — the large muscles at the back of the thighs.

AEROBIC A.M. WORKOUTS

Even if your morning routine consists of just a 10-minute walk, you're going to find yourself more bright-eyed and bushy-tailed than you would without it. Your cobwebbed coworkers may look as though they've been rolled to work on a stretcher, doing all they can just to rub the sleep from their eyes, but not you. You're going to be alert and ready to dig in because you've primed your body with oxygen. You've also worked out some morning stiffness and gotten your body's mood-elevating endorphins flowing to put you in a positive and productive frame of mind.

With aerobic exercise, especially, research shows that the body benefits most when exercise is done *comfortably*, not between gasping breaths. There's a time-tested rule of thumb regarding the optimal pursuit of aerobic endeavors that states that if you cannot comfortably converse with someone while you're exercising aerobically, it's not aerobically that you're exercising. You're exercising anaerobically, which means without oxygen, and therefore calling on different energy-producing mechanisms entirely.

But enough science. It's time to rise and get rolling.

Indoor 10-Minute A.M. Aerobic Workouts

Feel free to watch television or listen to the radio while doing these activities, of course, and as for clothing to wear — think simplicity and speed: Even your pajamas or underwear will do just fine.

Jumping jacks. This is a great workout, but be sure your floor is sturdy so you don't disturb your neighbors or rattle dishes off your shelves.

Rowing machine. With the right machine (you get what you pay for) rowing can be a great exercise for building strength as it also works the cardiovascular system.

Skipping rope. An excellent workout that takes little time, but, again, do it only on sturdy flooring.

Stair-climbing using machine. Another good cardiovascular workout, and one that lets you catch the morning news.

Stair-climbing using real stairs. It's cheaper and just as effective as the new gizmos.

Treadmill. Great for walking or running or a combination of both.

Running in place. If you run at a moderate pace, you can cover a mile or more in 10 minutes.

Stationary bike. Your quads will thank you for time spent on this machine. Make sure the one you choose has a comfortable saddle and isn't too noisy.

Step aerobics. One of the best cardiovascular workouts

around. Good strengthener for legs and arms, too, if arm movements are employed.

10 minutes of a video workout. Choose a good 10-minute segment — or tape part of your favorite TV exercise show.

Outdoor 10-Minute A.M. Aerobic Workouts

Just *getting* outside in the morning can be invigorating, but 10 minutes of exercise will really get you going. If any of the following suggestions might be disruptive to the particular attire and/or hairstyle your job requires for the day, however, you can always opt for an indoor workout instead. Switching between the two types of workouts can add a nice variety to your morning pursuits, in fact.

Walking your dog. A dog is great incentive to get you out in the morning, but you can just as easily squeeze in a 10-minute walk without one, too.

Jogging or running for 10 minutes. Running is one of the most calorically costly exercises you can do. Be sure to have good shoes, and expect some soreness in the first few weeks.

Walking for 10 minutes after parking. Park your car in the usual spot but walk for ten minutes before beginning your day.

Walking for 10 minutes after getting off the train, bus, or subway. Get off at your normal spot or a couple of stops early, and don't be afraid to bail out of that car pool several blocks early, either.

Riding a bike for 10 minutes — or all the way to work! If you go early enough, you'll miss the traffic. Otherwise, use side streets to play it safe.

Jumping rope. A five-minute session of outdoor rope jumping can give your cardiovascular system an invigorating workout. Rest when you need to, breathe through your

The Commuter's Workout

You can put your commuting time to work — with a little imagination — whether you're in a car, on a bus, or on a train. Isometric exercises, which use resistance to work muscles, are the way to do it.

Riding. If you're lucky enough to be a passenger, do as many of these simple exercises as time allows. If you're driving, do these only at a stop sign or red light, or at other times when your car is *not* in motion. (See Appendix A: the Exercises for illustrated instructions.)

- Isometric Curls
- Shoulder Rotations
- Neck Stretch
- Hip Switch with Neck Stretch
- Shoulder Stretch
- Chin Tuck

Driving: If you're the driver, the exercises you do must not in any way jeopardize your safety. The isometrics that follow will leave you free to drive and respond instantly to anything that develops on the road.

- Isometric tummy-tighteners: Contract the muscles of your abdomen for 10 seconds (as if someone were about to deliver a punch to that area), pressing your back against the seat. Hold for 10 seconds. Repeat for a total of 10.
- Isometrics also work well for your butt muscles. Tighten, hold for 10 seconds, and repeat for a total of 10.
- Work your thigh muscles (quadriceps) with isometrics, too. Tighten, hold for 10 seconds, and repeat for a total of 10.

Don't forget to use your imagination to think of new ways to get fit as you commute. Listening to music, too, can inspire you to get moving — even if it is just one muscle at a time.

nose, and land as lightly as possible on the balls of your feet.

Swimming. This is a great calorie-burner, plus it's just what the doctor ordered for most people who suffer from back pain.

STRENGTH WORKOUTS FOR THE A.M.

Remember, your daily goal is to get at least 20 minutes of cardiovascular exercise, 5 to 10 minutes of strength activity, and 5 to 10 more minutes of stretching, divided into whatever increments and accomplished at whatever times you find most convenient. So if it's some mild grunting and groaning you might prefer to do before beginning your day, try any of the following. And again, no elaborate exercise attire required. Flannel pajamas will absorb a little morning perspiration as well as any sweat suit.

Indoor Strengthening Exercises

Before you shower, try spending 5 to 10 minutes doing these strengtheners. (See Appendix A for illustrations of these exercises and more.)

Back and Butt Builder. This exercise feels like swimming on land and can be done before you even get out of bed.

1. Lie facedown with your feet slightly apart and your arms stretched out in front of you.
2. Keeping your head down and your abdominal muscles tightened, lift one leg and your opposite arm 6 to 12 inches off the floor. Hold for at least 5 seconds. Repeat for a total of 10, then switch to your other arm and leg for 10.

Semi Sit-ups. Another good in-bed exercise, this one tightens the abdominals. Keep your arms straight out in front of you, crossed over your chest, or with hands clasped behind your neck, depending on your level of fitness.

1. Lie on your back with your legs bent. Keeping your chin tucked, raise your head and shoulders.
2. Hold for 5 seconds and slowly lie back down. Do 3 sets of 10: one forward, one to the right, and one to the left.

Arm Curls. If you have 1- to 3-pound weights, use them for these exercises. If you don't, use cans of soup or jars of spaghetti sauce.

Wall Slides. Nothing beats this exercise for firming upper thighs.

1. Stand against a wall with your feet about a foot from it. Keep your feet about a foot apart.
2. Slide down until your knees are bent at a 90° angle. Hold for a count of 10 and repeat as many times as you can.

Toe Raises. A good calf firmer, this can be done most anytime of the day.

1. Raise both heels from the floor to stand tip-toe. Hold for a count of 5.
2. Lower and repeat 10 times.

Isometric Curls. While waiting for your coffee to brew, do 3 sets (10 repetitions per set) with a 1-minute rest in between.

1. Clasp your hands together in front of you with your elbows bent at about a 90° angle. The palm of your right hand should be facing upward, the palm of your left hand, downward.
2. Lift upward with your right hand will all the force you can while pushing down with your left hand. Hold for about 5 seconds with your hands remaining essentially motionless.
3. Repeat with hands in opposite positions.

A WORD FOR ARTHRITIS SUFFERERS

If you suffer from arthritis, you have yet another reason to work your workouts into your morning routine: Exercise, and stretching especially, can help alleviate stiffness in joints, which tend to tighten up as we sleep. I can vouch for this personally, as an old football injury has left me with a pretty nasty case of arthritis in my lower back that leaves me feeling about as mobile as a mannequin when I first roll out of bed. After several minutes of stretching, however (pulling my knees into my chest is especially effective), followed by some chin-ups and a quick aerobic workout on my rowing machine, I feel like a new guy.

Exercise can help soothe painful arthritic joints not only by "greasing" them with a natural lubricant known as synovial fluid, but by strengthening the muscles that support them, thereby protecting the joints by absorbing impact in ways that weaker muscles could not. "By strengthening the muscles around a joint," says George E. Ehrlich, M.D., director of the Division of Rheumatology at Hahnemann Hospital and Medical College in Philadelphia, "you not only help protect the joint, you allow it to function as it was designed."

Check first with your doctor before you start exercising if your condition is serious. It's going to be my guess, however, that you'll be getting a green light, and a very enthusiastic one.

PUTTING IT ALL TOGETHER

Early morning exercise is such a great eye-opener because it's such a great artery-opener, providing your body's cells with the oxygen and other vital nutrients they need to come to life after a night's sleep. The lift that morning exercise gives you comes from the mood-boosting cocktail of endorphins, which can produce a first-grade "high" with no strings attached, except better health.

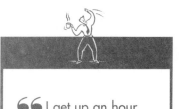

> 66 I get up an hour before anyone else in my family so I can exercise in peace. After about 30 minutes of working out, I fit in 20 minutes of meditation. I've been doing this for years, and it's become my favorite part of the day. 99
>
> JIM, librarian

Even if your morning routine is just some jumping jacks and light stretching in the shower, it's going to make a noticeable difference in how you feel, mentally as well as physically — precisely the stuff of which career advancement is made, according to Robert K. Cooper, author of *Health and Fitness Excellence* and *The Performance Edge*. For most of us in today's hyper-automated world, "increasing our physical activity is the single most important thing we can do to improve the way we look, feel, think and perform," according to Dr. Cooper. Better yet, it doesn't take a lot of effort to bring these energizing changes into play.

So try to make at least some form of exercise a regular part of your morning routine. And if none of the workouts we've suggested seem to be your style, come up with one of your own. No one knows your schedule, your *body*, or your temperament better than you do, after all, so you be the fitness instructor. Be creative and be flexible, varying your activities as circumstances dictate, but always remembering that exercise is exercise whether it's done in a sweat suit or your birthday suit, in a health club or on your bedroom floor. You'll be burning calories and building health the same as any fitness guru with chrome barbells and a full-length mirror.

Making Fitness Fit
On the Job

W ork. Boy, has that word been redefined over the years. What used to require two arms and two legs now requires little more than something to sit on. At the beginning of this century, more than 30 percent of the energy needed to run the U.S. economy came from the power of human muscle, but today that figure has dwindled to less than 1 percent. For all the good technology has done, it also has turned some broad shoulders into bay windows and size 8s to size 12s.

If this rings true you might think about employing the hours between 9 and 5 for physical as well as fiscal ends, for the good of your health, your physique, *and* your career.

Utterly impossible, you say? You're desk-bound, phone-bound, and computer-bound to boot?

Not to the degree you think. Besides, even if you can manage to burn only an additional 100 calories at work per day, that's still two-thirds of the minimum daily requirement of 150 calories needed to satisfy your 1,000-calorie-a-week quota. *And* it's enough to burn off seven pounds of fat in a year!

But perhaps best of all — and this is what many people wind up liking most about getting more exercise at work —

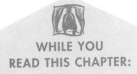

**WHILE YOU
READ THIS CHAPTER:**

Do Shoulder Rotations with right shoulder, then your left.

it's on company time! That's right, you will be getting *paid* to get fit, which you should feel free to consider the greatest perk of all in this deal. Our profit-minded companies are the ones that took workplace exercise away from us in the first place, after all: Why shouldn't they allow us to take some of it back?

Could you be heading toward a pink slip with the sort of workplace workouts I have in mind? Not if you behave yourself. The activities I'll be suggesting, by making you more energetic and alert, may even help *further* your career. Research shows that exercise is a significantly better energizer than the likes of a pastry or a candy bar, so by pursuing fitness on the job, you just might also be pursuing a raise.

These same energizing effects can also be enjoyed by all of you who work at home, of course, perhaps even more so because you're limited by fewer "managerial" constraints. By building short periods of exercise into your day, you'll have more energy, you'll be more alert, and you'll also find yourself more resilient to the stress of dealing with children that — sorry, all you CEOs — can make the workplace seem like a retreat.

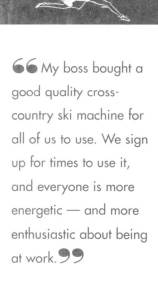

66 My boss bought a good quality cross-country ski machine for all of us to use. We sign up for times to use it, and everyone is more energetic — and more enthusiastic about being at work. 99

SALLY, office manager

COFFEE BREAKS WITHOUT CAFFEINE

Getting fit on the job sounds great, but you're going to have to see it to believe it, right?

Then let's start with the coffee break — that coveted workplace institution whereby we attempt to derive energy from caffeine and/or calorically catastrophic pastry. A little high-octane java and maybe a cream-filled doughnut or two and you're back in the saddle. Sound familiar?

Careful. The intentions of the coffee break may be good, but its effects all too often are not. Studies show that caffeine, especially in combination with snacks high in sugar (such as a croissant or a candy bar), can create a situation surprisingly illustrative of Newton's third law of motion: What goes up must come down. Blood sugar rises so fast in response to the sugar/caffeine combo that the pancreas panics, putting out enough insulin to cause a severe blood sugar *drop*. The result can be light-headedness and lethargy, which many of us try to remedy, unfortunately, by partaking of more of the very culprits that clobbered us in the first place.

The natural energizer. That's not so, however, with exercise! Exercise energizes *naturally* by summoning blood sugar (glucose) from the liver at a rate the pancreas can live with. The result is a more subtle but *lasting* energy boost not followed by the sort of crash caused by the likes of a blueberry Danish and cappuccino. Exercise also decreases your craving for that snack. Considering all the other benefits of exercise (see chapter 2), you'd have to be a little nutty *not* to consider it as a midmorning boost. Why *consume* calories for energy, after all, when you can *combust* them instead?

Please consider these midmorning energy-boosters with that in mind. Followed by some fruit juice and/or a low-fat snack such as yogurt, rice cakes, or whole-grain bread, they just might help improve your productivity along with your health.

Cardiovascular exercise is great as a midmorning boost because it infuses the body with energizing oxygen, helps remove waste products that have accumulated in the blood, and roots out the kinks that are the bane of the desk-bound life. Try one of the following with these *natural* perks in mind.

 A 10-minute walk in the parking lot, or up and down your company's corridors.

 Ten minutes of climbing stairs. (There must be some in the building somewhere.)

 Several minutes of jumping jacks in your office if you have one, in the rest room if you don't.

 Running in place for 5 minutes. Take 30-second rests each minute if need be.

Or if your company has a fitness center within quick enough reach:

 Several minutes of stationary cycling. (One enterprising woman I know brought her own to use in the office.)

 Several minutes of walking or slow running on a treadmill.

 Several minutes of rowing on a rowing machine.

Strength-building exercises also can be energizing and have an advantage over some of the above cardiovascular activities by virtue of not demanding as much space. Several of these, in fact, you can do right at your desk.

 Isometric Curls* for the biceps and triceps can be done anywhere.

 Curls can also be done with resistance supplied by your desk.

 Wall push-ups are great for those upper arm muscles.

Chin-ups are great for those who have already developed arm muscles. (A chin-up bar is necessary for these, of course, but all you need for installing a portable model is a stable doorway.)

 Forward lunges can be done at your desk.

 Lumbar stabilization exercises such as the Quadriped* help combat desk fatigue.

Flexibility exercises are just what muscles need after several hours of being sequestered behind a desk, sales counter, or steering wheel. Try these for giving muscles a second wind.

 Shoulder Rotations* relieve your shoulders and neck of the stress that builds up all day. Create as much movement in your upper back muscles as you can while you do them.

 The Reach* can be done standing or sitting. Stretch your hands as high above your head as you can while taking a deep breath. Hold for about 5 seconds, then exhale as you lower your arms.

 The Neck Stretch* will relieve your neck and upper back of stress. Simply tuck your chin into your chest. If you like, gently tip your head to the left, return to center, then tip to the right.

 Arm Circles* are good to do whenever you're standing. Hold your arms straight out from your sides. Move them in circles, increasing the size with each circle. Do about 10 in each direction.

 The Upper Back Bend feels great after sitting for a while. Clasp your hands behind your neck and gently lean back in your chair as far as possible. Open and close your mouth to stretch the jaw muscles, then slowly sit back up.

 The Lower Back Stretch* relieves pressure on the lower back. While seated, grasp your right knee and slowly pull it up into your chest as far as possible while you keep your other leg straight. Hold for about 5 seconds, and then do the same with the other leg.

See Appendix A for instructions and illustrations.

EXERCISE AT YOUR DESK

Most of us think of sitting as effortless, but that's not how the typical office worker who's been stuck at a desk in front of a computer feels after eight long hours. Though the calorie expenditure isn't equal to some more rigorous blue-collar endeavors, sitting imposes tremendous stress on the back and does nothing to aid circulation. So how can we earn our paychecks and fit fitness in at the same time? Again, it's all in the mind.

Remember to move: That's the key to working out at your desk. While it's advisable to get up and walk about every 30 minutes or so, you won't need to do that so often if you incorporate a few simple yet extremely beneficial exercises into those hours at the desk. Movements that refresh the body with oxygenated blood and relieve muscles and joints through stretches will serve the same purpose as a spirited walk around the block. Many of these movements can be done so inconspicuously, moreover, that no one need know that you're doing them. Besides, even if your movements do catch the eye of a befuddled onlooker, all you have to do is be honest about what you're up to. Clue your coworkers into what you're doing and why, and maybe suggest that they adopt a few of your moves themselves. Who knows, your entire office soon could be into your "desk-ercise" habit, enjoying a marked improvement in fitness as well as efficiency as a result!

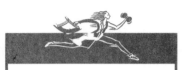

> 66 I never felt comfortable doing stretches at my desk when I was in plain view of everybody else in my office. I'd always find some reason to get up so that I could stretch. Now that we have dividers, I can do stretching exercises without leaving my desk, even when I'm on the phone. Now I feel better, and I'm more efficient because of it. 99

NANCY, accountant

Desk Exercises

Relieving your body from the stress of sitting increases blood flow, energizes tired muscles, and makes you feel better and more alert. Try these stretches for a more comfortable — and productive — workday.

■ Move from side to side on your chair, raising your hip up toward your shoulder, alternating left to right. This stretches your back, hips, and shoulders.

■ Keeping your back straight and your arms on the armrests of your chair, lift your foot until your leg is straight and, breathing, hold it for a few seconds. Repeat with the other leg, remembering to keep your back straight. You should feel a good stretch behind your knees.

■ Roll your shoulders, one at a time.

■ Push your chest forward and bend your head back, causing your back to arch. Then do the opposite movement: Roll your shoulders forward and lower your chin to your chest as you round your back. Repeat.

■ If you hold the telephone between your shoulder and your ear, be sure to do so on the opposite side periodically to stretch the muscles that were contracted and contract the muscles that were stretched.

■ Raise your arms in front of you and clasp the wrist of one arm with the hand of the other. Pull forward on the wrist for a good stretch. Reverse.

■ Raise your arms above your head and clasp the wrist of one arm with the hand of the other. Pull up. Reverse.

■ If you don't mind a few stares, or if you have a private office, give yourself a good hug. Wrap your arms around your torso and twist slightly from side to side.

■ Chin tucks (as described in Appendix A) are a wonderful way to stretch the neck and shoulders as well as to train your body to maintain good posture. Get in the habit of doing a chin tuck every time you stop typing (or start a new paragraph or open a particular drawer).

■ Raise your right arm so that it's angled to the left. Cup your left hand under your right arm just above the elbow. Pull your right elbow toward your left shoulder for a half-hug and a good stretch. Reverse.

Some Quick Lessons on Sitting

It may sound silly that there could be room for improvement in something as basic as sitting, but for most of us there is, and especially if our jobs demand that we sit for extended periods. By sitting improperly, in fact, we risk draining ourselves of much of the energy our fitness efforts give us. It's like trying to store water in a leaky bucket. Here are some tips for putting an end to poor sitting habits — and making your chair time the restorative experience that it should be.

1.   **Don't slump.** "Sit as upright as possible, trying to keep as much of your back in contact with the back of your chair as you can," Dr. Cooper says. "Slouching or hunching over not only restricts breathing, but also impedes circulation and may put undue pressure on the heart." It also can increase pressure on the discs of the lower back by as much as 15-fold, studies show.

2.   **Don't cross your legs.** "Not only does crossing your legs choke off blood flow to the calves and feet, but it also can misalign the pelvis and put extreme pressure on the lower back," Dr. Cooper says. The best place for your feet is flat on the floor, or for variety you can put one foot ahead of the other in a slightly raised position on several phone books or a small stool. "If you must cross your legs," says Dr. Cooper, "do so only at the ankles."

3.   **Opt for a chair with armrests.** Studies show they can reduce pressure on the lower back by as much as 25 percent. They also alleviate pressure (pulling) on shoulders and neck.

4.   **Stop sitting on your wallet.** "Or on your checkbook, car keys, or anything else that could be tipping your pelvis," Dr. Cooper says. A study reported in the *New England Journal of Medicine* several years ago found that many low-back-pain sufferers were able to eliminate their back pain entirely just by emptying the contents of their rear pockets.

5.   **"Do not sit for more than 30 minutes at a time,"** Dr. Cooper advises. Get up and move around for at least 60 seconds — not just your comfort but also your ability to concentrate should be enhanced measurably if you do.

THE UPSIDE OF INTERRUPTIONS

If you're like most other people, you don't especially appreciate the interruptions that require you to get up from your desk, whether it's to retrieve a printed document, sign for an express package, or deliver a message. These interruptions can really get annoying and sometimes even cause us to get irritable. Why can't somebody else do it?

The modern way of thinking about fitness may change all that. Rather than regarding a trip downstairs to the fax machine as a time-wasting frustration, start seeing it as an opportunity to fit in some exercise — and on company time! The new attitude toward what you're doing will show, and your sunnier disposition will earn you compliments and maybe even a raise. Take a minute to deliver a letter to a colleague instead of relying on e-mail. And why not be the one to start a new pot of coffee when you finish off the last one? Bending over to get the coffee filter and pouch is great for flexibility. The next person who wants a cup will certainly appreciate your effort.

Build in a few stretches or strengthening exercises for every trip to the bathroom. You can do them in private and gain cumulative benefits that will soon be apparent. A good one for strengthening your quads is to slide your back down a wall until you're almost sitting, but without the chair. Hold that pose for 15 to 30 seconds and you'll feel the heat in your legs. Stretch your tired quads afterward: Grasp your heel behind you and pull your foot up to your behind, hold; then stretch the other side.

Creativity and imagination, you see, can aid your exercise efforts no matter where you are. You'll have more energy and whittle away that midriff bulge. Studies show that employees who are fit are more productive, so even your boss will be pleased. How can you go wrong?

Take a few minutes to deliver a message to a colleague instead of relying on e-mail.

EXERCISE FOR NON-DESK WORKERS

Those of us who work hard all day and don't get to sit much may feel no sympathy for the person sitting at a desk bemoaning that exercise is hard to come by. When your job has you on your feet all day, you may think you're getting *too much* exercise, and being "chained" to a desk might appear downright attractive. But don't think that just because you don't sit all day all of your basic exercise requirements are being fulfilled. Take a hard look at how your body moves throughout a typical workday and you may be surprised by what you find.

Workers whose jobs involve standing behind a counter know how exhausting not sitting can be, but standing in one place is not exercise. It's tiring and can cause real stress, especially to hip and back muscles. Exercise will be easier and equally as beneficial for you as it is for the office worker. Standees have the luxury of exercising their leg muscles almost as much as they wish, all the while earning their pay. Just browse through Appendix A for the exercises that fit your work environment and get busy!

If your job requires physical strength and activity, you probably don't need to fit more strength-building exercise into your workday. But you do need to train your body to move correctly to eliminate strain. The lumbar stabilization exercises in Appendix A are important for you to do. And don't think that lifting and exerting your body all day means that you don't need to improve your flexibility. Stretching is especially valuable when muscles are overworked. But you don't have to wait for a coffee break to do some stretching for a well-rounded workout. Incorporate it into the activities that are already part of your schedule. If you have to reach up to pound a nail, for example, be sure to stretch the opposite side afterward for balance. If you are painting a ceiling, always counteract the backward position of your head with a few Chin Tucks. And don't forget to include a few Shoulder Rolls.

LUNCH: REMEMBER THE SIDE ORDER OF OXYGEN

Twelve noon. Time for . . . the usual tuna sandwich and rice pudding from the company cafeteria? Lunch out somewhere with coworkers? Yogurt at your desk along with a juicy novel?

Whatever it is that you do for lunch, you can do more. Even if you get only 30 minutes instead of an hour, you can fit fitness into your lunch break. How long does it take, after all, to eat?

If you really need a full hour, I'm going to guess that might be one of your fitness problems right there. Yes, we should chew our food thoroughly, but that's a lot of food chewed.

The point is simply this: Today's lunch hour offers itself as one of the richest opportunities for exercise. Think about it:

1. *It doesn't dip into family time.* Don't you hate those dinners messed up by having to get to the health club, health-rider, fitness video, or whatever other nighttime exercise obligation you've come to despise?

2. *It can give you the energy you need when you need it.* And don't you regret those late-night workouts that rev you up only so you can stay up too late watching how to make fattening meals on the Food Network? Working out during lunch can juice you up for the rest of your *money-making* day.

3. *It can be free.* If your company has a fitness facility, and many do nowadays, some of those unaffordable exercise gizmos you lust for probably are there just waiting for you. And even if your place of business doesn't have a fitness facility, you'll be exercising on *company* time. Your lunch hour is built into your contract; you may use it however you see fit.

4.   It can put those lunch-time calories to work rather than just to fat. Sit back down at your desk after one of those four-star affairs intended to impress somebody, and what happens? Calories with nowhere to go generally turn to fat. But by working out — lightly — after you eat, you give all those chocolate mousse calories in your blood something more productive to do. Research shows that moderate exercise *after* eating, in fact, can increase calorie-burning by as much as 30 percent.

To Eat Before or After Exercise?

It's an often asked and very good question: When's the best time to eat in relation to noontime exercise?

Answer: That depends on the intensity of the exercise, and why it's being done. If your primary goal is to burn calories for the purpose of weight control, research shows it's best to eat before you exercise, so long as you're not going to be exercising too hard. By eating before you exercise, you increase what's known as the thermal effect of food. That means calories are more readily available for immediate use as fuel when consumed shortly before exercise. Food should be eaten within 30 minutes before exercise begins for this increased calorie-burn to occur, studies show, and the increase can be substantial — as much as 30 percent, in fact.

But if your reasons for exercising are more performance oriented — perhaps you'd like nothing more than to whip a colleague or two in the next corporate 5K — you'd do better to eat *after* your lunch-hour workout. The greater intensity with which you'll be exercising could cause digestive discomfort if you eat beforehand.

Tips for Lunch Time Fitness

You can get more out of your lunch break than food. With imagination and resourcefulness, it can be the key to fitting in fitness.

■ *If your company has a fitness room, for heaven's sake, use it.* Many corporate fitness facilities today rival even the finest health clubs, so you'd be silly not to cash in. For a cardiovascular workout, use either a stationary bike, stair-climbing machine, treadmill, rower, or cross-country skier. For a strength-building workout, use free weights (barbells and dumbbells) or one of those bizarre-looking weight machines (studies are equivocal about which of these two approaches is better, so let your preference be your guide). Ask the instructor at your facility for assistance in putting together a workout suited to your cardiovascular or strength-building needs, or see Appendix A and put together a workout on your own.

■ *Explore the great outdoors.* This may not be feasible in certain urban environments, but if your place of work is in a reasonably safe and natural setting, kick off your heels or wing tips, lace up your walking shoes, and get strolling. An advantage of walking for your lunch time exercise, as opposed to doing something more strenuous such as jogging or getting a tough cardiovascular workout at the fitness center, is that you can do it *after* you eat, thus boosting the number of calories you burn. You also spare yourself the time and trouble of having to shower.

■ *Explore the great indoors.* If weather conditions are unfavorable, or you simply don't like the locale of your place of work, stroll the corridors (if your complex is large enough) or head for the nearest mall. Maybe even do some quick grocery shopping while afoot on your midday spree. You'll be increasing the calories you burn by carrying those bags, and you'll save yourself from having to do it at night.

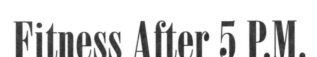

Fitness After 5 P.M.

Work is supposed to be *over* when you get home — time to relax and be with the family, to stretch out and catch up on the day, to unwind, not switch directly from your work clothes into a sweat suit.

True. But remember: If you've already been nibbling away at your DEA (Daily Exercise Requirements) in some of the ways recommended in this book, you won't need that sweat suit. If you've already managed to squeeze in two 10-minute cardiovascular workouts, in fact — one in the morning and one at lunch — you can consider anything else you do for the day to be icing on the cake.

Take the case of Paul. He gets a short walk in the morning and another one at noon; thus, his precious evening hours are open for any number of highly pleasurable activities involving his family or requiring his services around the house or yard.

"Some nights I'll take a walk with the kids to the park and get some strength exercise messing around with them on the jungle gym," he says. "Other nights I'll do something physical in the way of yard work, such as clipping hedges, working in the garden, cutting some grass, that kind of thing. Or if the weather's bad, I have a set of weights I'll push around for a while in

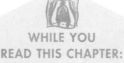

**WHILE YOU
READ THIS CHAPTER:**
Sitting up straight, tuck your chin back in line
with your torso. Hold and repeat every time you think of it.

the basement. I've gotten myself in the habit of always doing at least something, even if it's just helping my wife with some of the housework. She also works, so she really appreciates any help she can get."

Atta boy, Paul! Your fitness program certainly gets high marks.

"But best of all is the difference it's all made," Paul hastens to add. "What I'm doing hardly feels like any sort of structured program, yet I've lost close to 20 pounds in the past year, and I seem to have so much more energy."

Aha! Therein lies the secret of fitness when approached in the easy-does-it style I've been recommending since the opening pages of this book. When pursued at a pace the body finds comfortable, fitness begets fitness. The more active you are, the more active you will *feel* like being and your fitness level will spiral upward in an exponential fashion. A most *un*viscious circle.

"I used to get home from work and head straight for the TV, because I felt too pooped to do much else," Paul confesses. "But now I get home champing at the bit to get into one of the projects I've got going."

Handy and healthy. That's Paul. You don't have to be a Bob Vila to burn calories pleasantly and productively in your leisure hours, though. Consider Joan, a 36-year-old working mother of two, who also gets her evening exercise in fun and meaningful ways but wouldn't know a dovetail joint if it flew in her face.

"Two nights a week in the summer," says Joan, "I'm the manager of a softball team, which one of my daughters plays on, and I make sure to get plenty of exercise during our warm-ups for the games. We also practice on Saturdays, so I get another workout there. We all do stretching exercises together, and some running. It adds up to a pretty good workout."

With the turning of the leaves, Joan turns to coaching soccer, in which *both* her daughters participate. "I certainly get my cardiovascular workouts there," she says. "And not just during practices. Even during the games, I find myself running up and down the field to follow the play."

In the winter, Joan's fitness turns to coaching basketball. "I

> *The key to finding a leisure-time fitness activity you will not leave is finding a leisure-time fitness activity you can love.*

just love working with kids," she says. "They have such energy, and it's contagious. I find myself doing all this strenuous exercise, but it doesn't feel like exercise. I guess it's because I get so involved."

FITNESS FOR THE FUN OF IT

Beginning to see a pattern here? Paul can't wait to break a sweat with his next renovation project, climb on the jungle gym, or give an after-dinner piggyback at the request of his three-year-old. And as Joan says of her time running around like a teenager in her duties as a volunteer coach, "It's the most rewarding part of my day."

Which says it in a nutshell. Some people participate in a sport; others discover a hobby. Whatever it is, it should be something that satisfies you and that you actually look forward to doing. Fitness after 5 o'clock, in short, should be for the fun of it.

But nothing that comes even close to inducing a sweat could fill that bill, you say?

I challenge you to test that claim. Below are some ideas for leisure-time activities that are fully capable of providing substantial fitness and fat-burning benefits, yet would be very difficult, indeed, to classify as onerous:

If you have children, involve them. Take them for nature walks, or even just walks to the nearest ice cream store if you live in the city (and don't worry, you'll have earned yours). Or do sporting activities with them — play whiffle ball, Frisbee, tennis, badminton, even horseshoes or croquet. You'll at least be doing more than watching *Wheel of Fortune*, and you'll also be getting your children into the healthful pattern of being active — very important for influencing their exercise behavior as adults, studies show.

If you own a home, improve it. And don't worry if you know as much about dovetail joints as Joan. Hoodwink a friend who does know, and work along as a helper. Or hire a professional if no such friend exists, and work along on weekends until you know enough to go it alone. (That's the way Paul got started. He took his vacation one summer to work alongside the carpenter

Calorie-Burners

Any activity can qualify as exercise, but to burn your 1,000 to 2,000 calories per week, you might want to add some that burn calories faster — especially if time is at a premium.

| ACTIVITY | CALORIES/MIN. | | | |
	120 LB.	140 LB.	160 LB.	180 LB.
Basketball	7.5	8.8	10.0	11.3
Bowling	1.2	1.4	1.6	1.9
Cycling (10 MPH)	5.5	6.4	7.3	8.2
Dancing (aerobic)	7.4	8.6	9.8	11.1
Dancing (social)	2.9	3.3	3.7	4.2
Gardening	5.0	5.9	6.7	7.5
Golf (carry/pull clubs)	4.6	5.4	6.2	7.0
Golf (power cart)	2.1	2.5	2.8	3.2
Hiking	4.5	5.2	6.0	6.7
Jogging	9.3	10.8	12.4	13.9
Running	11.4	13.2	15.1	17.0
Sitting (quietly)	1.2	1.3	1.5	1.7
Skating (ice and roller)	5.9	6.9	7.9	8.8
Skiing (cross country)	7.5	8.8	10.0	11.3
Skiing (water and downhill)	5.7	6.6	7.6	8.5
Swimming (crawl, moderate pace)	7.8	9.0	10.3	11.6
Tennis	6.0	6.9	7.9	8.9
Walking	6.5	7.6	8.7	9.7
Weight Training	6.6	7.6	8.7	9.8

Source: American Council on Exercise

building his deck and learned enough to remodel his family room. Not only did he lose five pounds during those two deck-building weeks, but he also saved himself about $400!)

If you're a competitive type, compete. Sports can be especially suitable for those of us who inherently seem to get ourselves too busy, because they can help channel the aggression that makes us overbook ourselves in the first place. Besides, activities such as tennis, softball, racquetball, and squash can be great exercise as well as fun. Why come home and crunch more numbers when you can crunch the likes of a tennis ball instead? Research confirms that we aggressive types do best when we let our aggressions out, so we'd be foolish not to do so in ways capable of bettering our health along the way.

If you like animals, show it. Amazing but true: Studies show that pets can help us live longer; they are sources of comfort more important than we realize. So what better way to grab a few extra years than by taking Fido for more of those walks he craves? Or even Morris? Undertake the care and riding of something as large as a horse, and you could really have some exercise on your hands. As the American Council on Exercise poster that pictures a dog states, "Think of him as an exercise machine with hair."

If you like vegetables, grow them. How many avid gardeners do you know looking plumper than their tomatoes? Not many, and the reasons are simple: Vegetables are virtually fat-free, and gardening can make for some awesome exercise. The digging builds cardiovascular endurance as well as muscular strength, and the weeding and picking are great stretching movements. Start delivering all those extra tomatoes to neighbors by *foot*, and you'll really have a victorious garden on your hands.

If you like dancing, just do it. Dance instruction has come a long way since Arthur Murray taught the tango. There's now improvisational jazz dance to be learned, disco, ethnic, and of course square dancing and ballet, in addition to the ballroom types that Arthur stepped so well. So if you like to move to rhythms — which a lot of us do, as demonstrated by all the Walkmans we wear — dance is the best way to do it. It also can be a real sweetheart of a calorie-burner, as the physiques of the great dancers attest. Not just Arthur Murray, who was certainly no Humpty Dumpty, but Juliet Prowse, Fred Astaire, Ray Bolger, Rita Moreno, Rudolf Nureyev, and Gregory Hines.

If you like to shop, head to the mall. The number of miles you walk in just a few hours at a mall might surprise you. Check with the facility nearest you about a mall-walking program. Many malls open early in the day so that walkers can use the facility regardless of the weather. It's a great way to window-shop while getting an aerobic workout, and you can do it at your own pace — with no traffic.

If you like to visit with a friend, plan a walk. Walking and talking go together. For one thing, you have relative privacy if just the two of you are taking your daily constitutional together — no kids or spouse or nosy neighbors to interrupt. Another good reason for a walking visit is that it makes conversation feel more natural, since you're not facing each other. Some people feel less self-conscious talking about personal issues when they combine it with walking. Best of all, you're getting in some great exercise while strengthening your friendship.

If you love nature, go for a hike. Many communities have hiking clubs with weekly scheduled walks led by knowledgeable guides. But you can find your own path by seeking out bird or wildlife sanctuaries or state forests and parks. A day spent at a forest or on a mountain provides rejuvenation of the spirit as well as the body.

If you want to watch TV or a video, exercise at the same time. Get in the habit of doing some flexibility or strengthening

66 With such a packed schedule, I find it hard to keep in touch with my friends — and I do value their friendship. One of the best ways to catch up and have a good old heart-to-heart is by planning a walk, usually for a weekend morning when there are few other demands. What a pleasure those walk/talks are! 99

PATRICIA, psychologist

exercises whenever you watch TV, and your couch-potato days will be a thing of the past. You'll enjoy the show, benefit physically, and feel virtuous, all at once.

If you enjoy reading, go to a library or bookstore and work out as you browse. Think of scrutinizing those stacks as great opportunities for stretching and squatting. You'll feel a tremendous benefit all over if you pay attention to your movements as you look for the next good read.

If you crave speed and thrills, try in-line skating. It's excellent for strengthening and cardiovascular conditioning, but be sure to wear a helmet and elbow and knee pads for those unexpected spills.

FITNESS FOR TWO

Exercise, as you can see, takes many forms and appeals to many temperaments. It clearly is *not* for masochists only, as the no-pain, no-gain philosophy of the early aerobic era wanted us to believe. No, our hedonistic sides can head us in the direction of greater fitness quite nicely, in fact, as the bodies of most avid surfers, rock-climbers, cross-country skiers and backpackers show. It's far easier to burn calories while having *fun*, after all, than it is while swimming in pain.

So potentially pleasurable is the pursuit of fitness, in fact, that it can be courted even on dates — dinner engagements, no less. Follow a romantic meal with a romantic walk through a lighted park area, perhaps, or to a nearby movie theater, or maybe meander through a museum. You'll be boosting the rate your body burns off the calories from your meal, remember, by as much as 30 percent.

Or try a bicycle built for two. Cycle before your dinner or after your dinner or both. Or incorporate your cycling as part of an afternoon picnic.

The best way of all to burn calories as a couple, of course, is on the dance floor. Disco, ballroom, square dancing, the polka — take your pick. Depending on the amount of passion you employ, some steps can have you burning 400 calories an hour — more than jogging! No wonder Michael Jackson is such a stick.

FITNESS IN THE TUB

When all is said and done, possibly the most Epicurean arena for exercise is the bathtub. Get some bubbles going, maybe

Tub Stretches and Strengthening Exercises

The hot water of a bath can make "tubbing" ideal for stretching.

- Gently pull your right knee in as close as you can to your chest, hold for several seconds, then repeat with the other knee. (This is good for stretching the muscles at the back of the upper leg — the hamstrings — plus those troublesome muscles of the lower back.)

- Grab your right wrist with your left hand, raise your hands over your head, then lean slowly from side to side as far as you can, concentrating on stretching the muscles of your shoulders and neck. Switch your grip and repeat.

- Lean as far forward as you can, keeping your legs straight, and grab your toes. Hold for several seconds, then release. (This stretches the lower back, the hamstrings, and the calves.)

You can also do some strength training in the tub, if you're in the mood:

- Place your palms on the rim of both sides of the tub, and press yourself upward until your arms are straight. Lower yourself, then repeat until fatigued. (Good for the triceps — the muscles at the back of the upper arm — and also the chest muscles, or "pecs.")

- With legs slightly bent, grab behind your knees and try to pull your knees into your chest, providing resistance, however, so that you feel considerable tension in your forearms and biceps. Hold this position of exertion for about 6 seconds, relax, then repeat until you've done a set of 10.

some scented oils, a candle, who knows — maybe even an exercise partner (the size of your tub and energy levels permitting).

Assuming a solo experience, however, try some of the suggestions given on page 67. They come recommended by Carolyn Maxwell, who after a day of being chef, manager, bookkeeper, and sometimes bottle washer at her own restaurant admits she can begin to feel a little sautéed herself. "Especially nice about the bathtub workout, in addition to being so relaxing," she says, "is that you needn't follow it with a shower."

Fitness Around the House

What has four walls, a roof, a yard, and more opportunities for exercise than any health club this side of Muscle Beach?

That's right, the average American house. Between the sweeping, scrubbing, painting, polishing, pruning, washing, weeding, mopping, mowing, hoeing, and hammering, it offers exercise for every muscle in the body.

But are we capitalizing on all the heart-healthy and muscle-building activities our homes have to offer?

More and more we are not, surveys show. Where we could be burning calories, we're increasingly choosing to burn cash instead. We spent an incredible $14.2 *billion* in 1995 for lawn-care services alone, according to a recent Gallup poll. That averages out to a whopping $710 per household, good for an increase of 5 percent over the year before. This increase has been great for the likes of Lou's Lawn n' Leaf, of course, but not so great for our physiques. Our hedges, unfortunately, are now trimmer than we are.

The idea of getting exercise while building equity in our homes seems to have escaped us. We've been getting, or at least trying to get, our exercise in far more difficult and impractical

**WHILE YOU
READ THIS CHAPTER:**
Sit in a chair with feet flat on the floor.
Raise your right foot until your leg is horizontal. Hold for
a few seconds and slowly release. Repeat with your left foot.

ways. Consider Rita, for example, who hires a gardener and a baby-sitter so she can drive 25 minutes to her fitness club to do squat-thrusts, bent-leg sit-ups, and lat pull-downs to the tune of $40 a month. She also pays a valet parking fee to save herself from walking the few blocks that would be required if she parked on the street.

Or how about Chuck, who pays his neighbor's son to cut the grass while Chuck attempts to get back into the running program that earned him a spot (20 years ago!) on his college track team. If he's not in his podiatrist's office, he's on crutches. Very rarely is he actually out on the road, as his 200 pounds sadly attest.

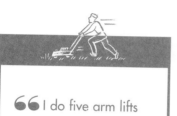

And then Lisa, who's been known to holler at her housecleaner not to run the vacuum while she's trying to exercise along with her favorite fitness show on TV! She used to do her own housecleaning, she confesses — when she wasn't so heavy. This is the same Lisa, incidentally, who recently was spotted taking the escalator instead of the stairs at a department store en route to checking out a fitness device that simulates — you guessed it — climbing stairs.

It's lunacy, but very few of us aren't guilty at least to some degree. We're having trouble getting over the fitness dictates of the past decades, which said, "Don the togs and heart-rate monitor or don't bother." That prescription squelched our hopes of getting any meaningful exercise puttering around our homesteads. We started looking at our household chores as more of a nuisance than ever because they didn't seem strenuous enough. Work around the house, we were led to believe, was something that only got in the way of working out.

> 66 I do five arm lifts with each grocery item weighing a pound or more as I put them away. For a ten-pound bag of potatoes, use both hands. For canned fruit use one in each hand. The big bag of dog food is really a challenge! 99
>
> MARTHA, corporate executive

Scientists have since found that notion to be all wet in its own sweat. Simply running the engine is what's most important; achieving high RPMs is needed only for those who want to get fit enough to win races or wear those T-shirts that stop at the navel. Remember, current research shows that most of us only need to supplement our normal lives with an extra 1,000 to 2,000 calories' worth of activity a week — whether it's by washing windows, painting shutters, or cleaning out the garage.

Get excited about bringing some of that wayward brawn of yours back to the home front, where it never should have left in the first place. Your house *has* missed you, you know — your multiple thumbs and all.

So come on back home, America! Your lawn, leaves, and leaking faucets forgive you and want you back. Start looking at your house or apartment not as a fitness enemy, but as a fitness ally. Whether it's a clogged drain, a hole in the roof, shutters that need paint, or backed-up rain gutters — it's *exercise*, a calorie-burner, a step toward a healthier heart and a longer life!

And don't overlook another eminently motivating reason to restock that tool kit of yours: the cents it can make. With the price of labor what it is these days, the money you can save by doing things yourself around the house could soon have your bank account as beefy as your biceps.

Thus, my nomination for Fitness Device of the Year — your home. What other gizmo allows you to expend calories so wisely? You don't just burn calories when you work around the house, you *invest* them. Your equity increases right along with your health, and you sure can't beat a fitness program like that.

1. ***Staple shut the Yellow Pages of your phone book.*** It's instinctive, isn't it? Something goes wrong with the toilet, or a board comes loose on the front porch, and bingo: You're into those Yellow Pages before you can say James Earl Jones. Break yourself of the habit. Invest in some books on home repair and learn to be more self-reliant around the house. Calories will be going up in smoke, not your cash.

2. ***Pretend you could be visited by your mother at any moment.*** This absolutely will keep you on top of things! Chores such as floor-scrubbing, vacuuming, and window-washing can be prolific calorie-burners — especially when done to the standards Mom would demand.

3. ***Know that a stitch in time saves nine.*** Try to be a little more vigilant about maintenance around the house. If the roof develops a small leak, fix it before it becomes a *big* one and *does* require professional care. The same with leaky faucets, chipping paint, and ominous-looking tree limbs. Learn to attend to things early rather than later, and your anxiety level (and possibly even your homeowner's insurance) will be lower right along with your cholesterol level and blood pressure.

4. ***Don't be afraid to do things the stupid way.*** You get paid to be smart at work, so at home you can afford to be a little dumb. Go ahead and leave a tool or two on the ground if you're working on the roof; the extra trips up and down the ladder will do you good. Cut the grass on gentle slopes by going uphill and down instead of sideways: a better workout for the legs. You get the idea. Your goal in puttering around the house shouldn't be efficiency, it should be e-fit-iency. You're out for exercise as much as you are to get stuff done.

5. ***Mean business when you work.*** More vigor means more fitness. Many house chores done with sufficient commitment can get your heart rate officially within its target zone (see page 26), which is the intensity sought by athletes in serious training. Besides, you'll finish sooner, and you have better things to do. Chores such as vacuuming, mopping floors, and washing windows can be done wimpishly or with gusto. Go for the latter.

6. *Involve the whole team.* Neatness is contagious. If you get neater, the kids will get neater, your spouse may get neater, and the result will be a neater ship in general — and, of course, greater energy expenditures will be needed to keep it that way.

7. *Go back in time.* Have to do the laundry? Hang it on the line instead of tossing it in the dryer. Time to bake a cake? Mix it by hand, not with the electric mixer. One of the chief reasons people struggle with their weight these days is that progress did away with these calorie-burning tasks. So bring them back: Imagine yourself living in the Little House on the Prairie if you have to. Every time you're presented with a chore, imagine how the Ingalls' family might have had to deal with it, and then give their method a try.

8. *Start watching some of those fix-it shows on PBS and cable TV.* You know, the ones you usually zoom right past on your way to *Melrose Place* or the ballgame. Well, don't. These shows can be quite engrossing, illuminating, and motivating. It helps to have an idea of what you'll be doing, after all, before you can feel frisky enough to go do it. You'll feel a great sense of satisfaction when you're done, and you'll also be fitter.

9. *Challenge yourself.* Take on something around the house that might be a little over your head. You'll learn from the experience, at least, and get fitter from it, definitely.

10. *Begin scheduling chores — and thinking of them — as real workouts.* Look at the calorie-burning charts on pages 63 and 75 and do a few quick calculations. As you can see, many household chores require all the same heart as more conventional exercise activities such as cycling, swimming, and even slow jogging. So place these chores on your schedule accordingly. You will not try to scrub the kitchen floor in addition to going to the gym on Tuesday night; you *will* scrub the kitchen floor *instead* of going to the gym Tuesday, and get a honey of a workout doing it.

JUST DO IT: YOUR WORK AND YOUR WORKOUTS, TOO

Here's a crash course in home maintenance, fat-fighting-style. Household chores are great calorie-burners and muscle-toners *without* any adjustments, of course, but by being aware of the possibilities for exercise when you do them, you can make them even better. Besides, in many cases these slight alterations can help you get your work done better and *faster* as well.

These tips focus on cleaning, but they can be applied to yard work and general repair around the house. And as much as some more traditional exercisers may scoff, work around the house — and yes, even cleaning! — will really provide exercise as worthwhile as that gotten in the gym. How else do you think Mr. Clean got to be such a hunk?

Push yourself. This needn't mean risking cardiac arrest, but it will mean putting some "heart" into your labor. Whether you're mowing the grass or making beds, you should work at a level of exertion that noticeably increases your rate of breathing but does not leave you so breathless that you could not comfortably converse with someone as you work. As with more traditional forms of exercise, this will ensure that you're giving your muscles enough oxygen to use fat as their primary energy source. By working *too* hard, you risk working anaerobically, which means you're exceeding your muscles' needs for the oxygen required to burn fat, forcing them to use the more easily burned glucose, a form of carbohydrate, instead.

Try to work continuously rather than in short spurts. Some research indicates that muscles need approximately a 10-minute warm-up period before doing their best fat burning, so try to pace yourself accordingly. Work hard enough so that you're breathing deeply, as explained above, but not so hard that you'll need to take breaks every few minutes.

Working around the house — even cleaning — can provide exercise as worthwhile as that gotten in the gym.

Household chores can be a great source of exercise. Use the following list for inspiration the next time you tackle a project, whether large or small. It all adds up!

CHORE	CALORIES BURNED PER HOUR*
INDOORS	
Ironing	120
Grocery shopping	175
Making beds	135
Mopping/sweeping	220
Painting	135
Putting groceries away	220
Scrubbing floors	400
Vacuuming	175
Washing dishes	120
Washing windows	250
OUTDOORS	
Carrying firewood	670
Chopping firewood (with ax)	360
Digging (with a pick and shovel)	585
Gardening (digging and hoeing)	460
Gardening (planting and weeding)	300
General carpentry	235
Mowing grass (with push-type rotary mower)	400
Painting (using a ladder)	315
Pruning trees (with handsaw)	475
Raking leaves	270
Sawing firewood (by hand)	465
Shoveling snow (powdery)	600
Stacking firewood	375
Trimming hedges (with manual clippers)	325
Washing/polishing car	225

*For a 150-pound person. Adjust caloric expenditures up or down slightly if you weigh more or less than this.

Target particular muscle groups. Different chores focus different muscles naturally, but you can gain even more benefit by sharpening this focus. When scrubbing a floor, for example, feel the tension in the back of your arms — your tricep muscles — and try to increase it (you'll be getting your floor cleaner, too). Employ the same strategy with sweeping, mopping, vacuuming, window washing, and scouring dirty dishes. All these activities employ specific muscles, which you'll be able to feel simply by paying attention. You can get a considerably better workout simply by applying a little more oomph.

Add auxiliary moves. Not all chores are inherently calorie-blasters, however, so some augmentation can be a good idea. When doing dishes or ironing, for example, try doing toe-raises to firm the muscles of your lower legs, or bun-tighteners (flexing the muscles of your posterior) to help bring up your rear. When vacuuming, give some extra work to your thighs by doing half-squats (bending at the knees to approximately a 90-degree angle). You can even get more muscular mileage out of washing windows by alternately holding the pail of detergent in your unoccupied hand, elbow slightly bent, to maximize benefits to your forearms and biceps.

In short, use your imagination to employ as much of your body as possible when you work. Do half-squats while raking leaves, and intermittent toe-touches while working in the garden. Learn to *think* of work around the house as a workout, in other words, and it will be.

> 66 I've trained myself to squat when I pick up my grandkids' things so that I'm strengthening my thigh muscles. I stretch my back when I bend over to unload the dishwasher, and I tighten my stomach muscles while I fold laundry. It might not seem like much, but it all helps. 99
>
> JANE, homemaker

Exercise "on" the House

There's exercise to be had not just "around" the house; there's exercise to be had literally "on" the house. Chores aside, your abode can be a veritable gymnasium if you know where to look.

Stairway push-ups. You can use any old flight of stairs (preferably carpeted) as a place to do inclined push-ups. They're identical to conventional push-ups except that you do them on an incline on your staircase rather than horizontally on the floor. This makes them somewhat easier than conventional push-ups, allowing you to do more.

Stairway calf stretches. Your stairs can also serve as an excellent device for exercising the calf muscles. Stand on the bottom step with your heels hanging off the edge. Lower and raise yourself, going down each time as far as you comfortably can. This is also great for stretching the Achilles' tendon (the large tendon that runs up the back of your lower leg starting at the heel). Do a set of 10 several times a day.

Porch dips. Your porch is also crying out to help you — provided its railing is sturdy enough. With your palms placed on the railing behind you, lower yourself as far as you comfortably can, then press up until your arms are straight again. This is an excellent strengthener for the chest muscles ("pecs") and triceps (at the back of your arms), which can swing as loosely as a hammock if neglected long enough.

Doorway deltoid strengtheners. Any doorway not busy with traffic can be an apparatus for developing the deltoids, the muscles at the very tops of your arms that give the shoulders more width. While standing in a doorway with your arms at your sides and the backs of your hands against the jambs, try to lift your arms upward and outward. Your arms won't go anywhere, of course, but that's the idea. You're working your deltoids isometrically. Hold each flex for about 6 seconds and repeat 5 times.

Kitchen chair step-ups. Even your furniture can get in to the exercise act, which you can discover by rethinking the chair. It's not just for sitting if it's unupholstered and stable enough: It can be used for developing the gluteus muscles, or "buns," if used as a tall step. Do a set of 10 such giant steps up and down from the kitchen chair, and you'll see. Very good for "bringing up the rear," indeed.

Fitness with (and for) the Family

Do you ever find yourself feeling guilty for exercising because it takes time away from being with your family? Then why not say "so long" to that guilt by inviting your family along whenever possible. Or maybe you could make efforts to join *them* in their fitness pursuits. The family that sweats together at least gets together, and that's a sizable portion of the communication challenge these days, is it not? Besides, in addition to facilitating your own fitness endeavors, you'll be aiding those of your fitness partners, as well, whether they be your children, spouse, or both.

But kids get enough exercise simply by virtue of being kids, you say? They're the last ones who need to worry about their fitness?

Unless your children are helping you run a several hundred-acre farm, that's unlikely to be true. Surveys show that our children are suffering from the same side effects caused by this hyper-automated society as we are. According to the American Council on Exercise, only 37 percent of children are considered physically active by the time they reach high-school age.

And don't think that just because your children are beyond an "impressionable" age that your attitudes about exercise no

**WHILE YOU
READ THIS CHAPTER:**
Clasp your hands behind you and straighten
your arms. Raise them and feel the stretch. Repeat.

longer affect them. "Whether we like it or not, our parental duty to serve as role models for our children is a lifelong affair," says psychotherapist Ronald Podell, M.D., author of *Contagious Emotions*. "Children are especially impressionable from early childhood through adolescence, of course, but they still look to us as examples once they're grown and may even have children of their own."

That's right, all you moms and pops. Your exercise obligations have just doubled. Not only do you owe it to yourselves to achieve a peaceful existence with exercise, but you owe it to your children as well. Think, for a moment, of the alternatives.

What, for example, might young Susie's chances be of developing a healthy relationship with exercise if she sees Mommy spending every spare moment on the couch in front of the TV munching corn chips? Or worse yet, Mommy grouchy and red-faced aboard some machine, "exorcising" more than exercising, searching for catharsis through sweat? Or how about Dad, who if not hobbling around on a bad knee caused by his training for a marathon is doing his imitation of Archie Bunker, beer in hand, married to his easy chair?

No wonder the fitness levels of our children are at an all-time low. We've been showing them exercise as something torturous or we haven't been showing it to them at all. Surveys show that approximately two-thirds of all children between the ages of 6 and 16 cannot even pass standard fitness tests given in school. Worse yet, an alarming 40 percent display a major risk factor

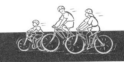

66 Before I got involved in sports myself, my kids gravitated toward the TV when they didn't have anything to do. I started working out — riding a bicycle and running — about a year ago, and now the kids want to go bike riding or run with me. They seem more interested in their general health, too — what they eat and how they take care of their bodies. **99**

JEFFREY, builder

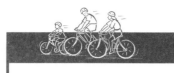

> 66 I never knew how difficult it is to hit a ball with a bat until I decided it was time for a mom to help coach Little League. I had a much better understanding of my daughter's feelings as she struggled to become a better hitter. My arm muscles improved, too. 99
>
> BARBARA, college instructor

for heart disease (high blood pressure, elevated cholesterol, or obesity) by the time they're — are you ready for this? — 8 years old!

At the rate things are going, the physical future of our children looks grim indeed. Studies have shown that three out of four children who remain obese through adolescence will be obese as adults. Couple that disconcerting statistic with surveys showing that childhood obesity currently is at an all-time high, and you can see why fitness educators are so concerned.

Johnny and Susie are not bionic. Much of the problem, of course, is that we think that youth is somehow impervious to the lifestyle onslaughts we struggle to avoid for ourselves as adults. Is it because we think that a diet of hot dogs and potato chips somehow gets turned into health food by some magical act of youth? Or that 25 hours a week of television (the national average for kids nowadays) somehow gets compensated for by a game of kickball once a week in physical education class?

The fitness and dietary standards we struggle to maintain for ourselves we somehow assume are unnecessary or possibly even harmful for our children. If you've ever bought your kids french fries and deep-fried chicken fingers at a fast-food restaurant while you've opted for the baked potato and broiled chicken fillet, you can see the irony.

We tend to treat our kids sometimes as if they were indestructible, but they are not. They're put together the same way we are, with the same hearts and arteries that can clog, and the same fat cells waiting to plump themselves up on excess calories if some sort of physical activity is not made available to intervene.

FITNESS LIKES COMPANY

Get the message? If there are children in your family, you're doing them what could be a long-term disservice by not helping them to establish a relationship with exercise conducive to making it a natural part of their lives. Before you get too depressed about that, however, consider the decidedly win-win situation this presents. If your children could use more physical activity — and you could, too — why, for Pete's sake, not join forces? The potential for symbiosis here is far too good to waste.

But more than just fitness can grow from joint-exercise ventures: There's also the emotional connection to consider. Time spent with our kids is time *invested* with our kids, as perhaps memories of your own childhood can attest. Mom and Dad showing the right way to swing a baseball bat or tennis racket is Mom and Dad showing they care.

And remember that whatever you can pull together will be miles better than nothing at all. As I've said more than once and in many ways, fitness can be a patchwork quilt of small and enjoyable efforts, not just a blanket of large and onerous ones. Whatever you can find the time to do with children, yours and other people's, will feel like a major change if you're currently doing nothing at all.

Encourage or Instruct Your Kids in Sports

Whether it's baseball, softball, T-ball, football, soccer, tennis, or anything else that gets those little bodies moving, just say yes. Parental encouragement — but not coercion — is important in helping children to make that often difficult first step into the athletic arena. Studies show that if children are not comfortable with their basic motor skills by the sixth grade, "they will never participate in physical activity as adults," says Paula K. Kun of the National Association for Sport and Physical Education. Encouragement from you as a parent, therefore, is important. Do be careful, however, as the dangers of being too forceful can equal those of not being forceful enough. Be sensitive to your children's athletic talents, or lack thereof, and be resourceful rather than derisive if it appears they may not have the gifts required to follow as deftly in your own athletic footsteps as you might like. I know one parent who decided, after her daughter's second month of tennis lessons, that life is too short for humiliation to that degree. She had a plywood backboard installed on the side of the garage so her daughter, with Mom's help, could practice in privacy. "We try to get out there at least a couple of times a week after dinner," Mom says. "And at the rate we're going, I think she's going to have a good shot at making her high school team, after all. Besides, I'm getting a nice workout, too."

It's a win-win situation, whether she ever wins an actual tennis match or not.

Encourage (and Participate in) Play

But there are certainly more ways to get and keep a little body fit than just through conventional organized sports. There's hide and seek, jump rope, hopscotch, Frisbee, whiffle ball, in-line skating, cycling, skateboarding, and climbing trees. And don't be shy about asking to tag along with your kids as you encourage them to pursue such activities. Do be prepared for some humiliation of your own, however, if you do. Any athletic glories you may have enjoyed in the past are unlikely to spare you from the rigors these "games" can demand.

A Pool for All Reasons

Sure, we all dream of the kidney-shaped in-ground pool, but children generally can have just as much fun, and get just as much exercise, splashing around in an above-ground pool — especially if you're in there splashing with them. Organize races by doing laps around the pool. They swim, you "run" — a fantastic workout for the legs, as you'll quickly find out.

Follow Your Hoop Dreams

Put up a basketball hoop for years of vigorous exercise for kids of all ages. A few games of one-on-one with a feisty teenager will show you both very quickly just what a "magic" form of exercise basketball can be.

Get in the Swing with a State-of-the-Art Play Structure

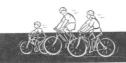

Have you seen some of the Taj Mahals now available? In a pinch you could live in one of them! But don't be swayed by the bells and whistles; the swings, climbing ropes, monkey bars, and sliding boards are what demand bodily exertion. And don't scrimp on quality. Not only will the unit be safer and last longer but you'll be able to be out there monkeying around on the thing (and getting a great strength workout) yourself.

Share the Health with Neighbors and Friends

If you don't have the space for creating a backyard of exercise opportunities yourself, consider joining forces with friends or neighbors in the name of fitness. Maybe the Joneses could handle the pool or the jungle gym if you offer your backyard for the badminton or volleyball net. Or perhaps organize a group within your community to build a state-

> 66 Children really enjoy the sense of accomplishment that comes from helping out, even if it's a small thing. They love the feeling of competence and involvement, especially if it's done with you. Whether it's helping with big tasks like raking leaves or little tasks like carrying out the garbage, it all contributes to a healthy self-esteem, as well as a healthy body. 99
>
> MARGARET, elementary school teacher

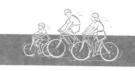

of-the-art playground that the entire neighborhood could use. (Considerable exercise would be in store for all those volunteering to help with its construction, too.)

Go on Walks with, and for, Mother Nature

In addition to being great exercise, walks with your kids can be a terrific experience. Depending on where you live and where you walk, you can discuss everything from the bees and the birds to . . . "the birds and the bees" if your children are of an age to be interested.

Or you can discuss, just as meaningfully, trash. Helpful in this regard is a little game to be played while depositing items of litter in plastic trash bags. Ask your kids to try to imagine the types of people responsible for these crimes against Mother Nature. Items such as beer cans, fast-food wrappers, and soda bottles should pose no great problem; those mattresses, refrigerators, tires, and fully loaded Hefty bags, however, might have you and your little ones scratching your heads.

Enlist the "Help" of Your Children When Working on the House or in the Yard

Granted, the help of a five-year-old when you're trying to put up a rain gutter or even just trim the hedges can be worse than no help at all — but that need not be true if you're willing to be a little creative. Consider Al, who achieved the seemingly impossible task of *productively* employing his four-year-old daughter for an entire afternoon while painting his garage. "I was using latex paint, so I gave her the job of priming the garage first with water. There was no way she could make a mess, and it really helped with what I was doing."

Nice job, Al. True usefulness aside, however, kids also can make great "gofers," as people who "go for" things are sometimes called. They can "go for" additional tools, even if you don't need them. Or they can go check what time it is, even if you're wearing a watch. Or they can go see if you've had any phone calls, even though you're not expecting any. They can go and get you some more lemonade, even though you may not be thirsty. So long as children are made to feel appreciated and important, they enjoy a sense of duty and accomplishment in doing nearly anything — and, of course, derive valuable exercise in doing so. Besides, their participation and companionship can be additional motivation for you to be more enterprising around the house and the yard.

Make TV-Viewing Special

This might not sound like an activity, but wait until you see the wrestling match that ensues. It's important that you come out on top, however, because surveys show that our kids now spend more time in front of the TV in a year's time than they do at school. Not only does that add up to a lot of inactivity, but it also adds up to a lot of very persuasive commercials for junk

It Hasn't Been Labeled the "Boob Tube" For Nothing

A study by the Harvard School of Public Health found a strong correlation not just between TV and unhealthful snacking but also between TV and obesity and between TV and poor performance in school.

foods. And if you've ever taken anyone younger than about 14 to the grocery store with you, you know the impact these ads can have. Worse yet, surveys indicate that kids tend to eat the foods they see advertised on TV as they're actually watching TV — double jeopardy.

So is it a total TV embargo you should enforce? No, because that's a wrestling match you probably would lose. Besides, there's some TV for kids that's educational, and some that's just good fun. Sit down with your kids and establish priorities. About 90 minutes a day, most experts agree, should be the limit, but don't feel you have to grant that much time in front of the tube. Some families ban TV-watching entirely during the week and allow selected shows on weekends. What's the result? Kids that start bouncing a basketball or reading a magazine when they have time on their hands.

Build a TV Alternative

Would your kids be glued to the idiot box if they had a treehouse, playhouse, or even a sandbox to entertain them? You have nothing to lose, except maybe a few pounds, by finding out. Get some plans from a hardware store or builder — or come up with a design of your own — and get hammering. Carpentry, depending on the fervor of your approach, can have you burning upwards of 1,000 calories in a four-hour (fun-filled) afternoon. It also can be a great way to interact with your young helper (or helpers) in an activity that employs brains as well as brawn.

WIN, DON'T LOSE, AN UNFIT SPOUSE

Your spouse is family too, of course, and as beneficial as fitness can be, surveys show that it can be a source of conflict between couples if each partner is not pursuing it at least somewhat equally.

It can be hard for both sides, says psychiatrist and author Thaddeus Kostrubala, for the fit and unfit partner alike.

"The pursuit of fitness can make profound changes in people," Dr. Kostrubala explains. "Usually these changes are for the good, but any time something is good for one member of a relationship without being good for the other, the potential for conflict exists."

Envy mixed with a sense of inferiority may begin to develop in the less-fit partner, according to Dr. Kostrubala, compounded by a growing sense of self-righteousness in the exercising partner. A wife who's getting fit and losing weight, for example, risks distancing herself from her husband if all he's doing is guiltily getting fatter every day on the couch. Of course, the reverse can be true: The husband who's out at the gym every night may not come home to warm embraces if his wife is feeling self-conscious and inferior for not following suit.

What can be done about these potential fitness conflicts? Exercise is tough enough to get without having to face emotional hurdles as well. A veteran of 27 marathons and three marriages himself, Dr. Kostrubala offers this advice:

1. If you're the exerciser and your spouse is not, encourage your spouse — as sensitively as possible — to join you in your fitness efforts. Walk together, cycle together, go to structured fitness classes together, exercise to a fitness video together — anything to get your spouse bitten by the fitness bug. Maybe even try something totally *new* together, such as tennis or golf, so the footing will be more equitable. If you can share in your spouse's clumsiness, the intimidation factor will be reduced substantially. Klutziness loves company just as much as misery does.

2. Talk honestly with your spouse about all the benefits of exercise — how it gives you more energy and more confidence in addition to the obvious perks of a trimmer and healthier body.

3. Plan fitness outings for the whole family — hikes, bicycle trips, golf junkets, canoe trips, doubles tennis (Mom and Dad vs. the kids, or other match-ups that might be more equitable). The more you can make fitness a family affair, the more it will make a positive and *lasting* impression on all concerned.

4. Tell your spouse you wish he or she would join you in your fitness pursuits so that you will not face spending your twilight years alone.

Fitness For the Road

E xercise is hard enough to find within the familiarity, comfort, and reasonable predictability of our own homes. So how in the name of Motel 6 are we supposed to find ways to exercise out there on the road? You know the scene: the cramped airline flights, slam-bam cab rides, drive-you-crazy hotel check-ins, and then that schedule of yours, packed tighter than your suitcase. It's almost impossible to find time for a shower, much less a workout.

Relax. I know personally every agony of which you speak. But as Francis Bacon had the wisdom to observe, "Adversity doth best discover virtue." You may have to learn to pack a portable chin-up bar along with your deodorant. Or stoop to doing jumping jacks for the first time since eighth grade. Or learn to work your "abs" while fending off the peanuts aboard Flight 102.

There's really just one basic rule for exercising on the road, you see: Do whatever you can, whenever you can, however you can, wherever you can.

Booking a room at a hotel with a decent fitness facility helps, of course, as does scheduling some time to use it, but unless you're Donald Trump, that's not likely to happen, especially if you're

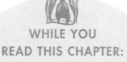

WHILE YOU READ THIS CHAPTER:
Sit straight and, pushing your shoulders back, squeeze your shoulder blades together. Hold and release. Repeat 5 times.

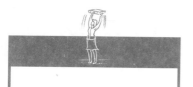

traveling on business and your company is cutting costs. No wonder the excuse is such a common one: "Sure, I'd like to get more exercise, but I'm on the road all the time. What am I going to do — carry barbells in my suitcase?"

As a matter of fact, that's a good idea (see "Secrets of a Superfit Salesman" on page 97), as is making sure to pack a jump rope in your carry-on bag.

Getting exercise on the road is no picnic, but then neither is traveling itself, so the nuisance of having to do a few jumping jacks here and there should fit right in. What difference is the inconvenience of a few makeshift calisthenics going to make?

Not a lot. Yet the difference such exercises can make in the way we *feel* when we're on the road can be huge. A several-hour plane flight, followed by a longer-than-expected layover, followed by another several-hour plane flight, followed by a wait for lost baggage, followed by a harrowing, New York City–type cab ride, may create a level of stress that few palliatives other than a good workout can relieve. (Several stiff cocktails at the hotel bar may be the more popular approach to mitigate such stress, but this usually just substitutes one set of problems for another, thus compounding a traveler's woes.)

It's cruel and unusual punishment, yes, but such is the way of flying the frenzied skies. We can go far, and we can go fast, but our minds and bodies pay for every mile. It's enough to make you wonder whether we did the right thing by demoting our horses and buggies in the first place.

Just as miserable is the family trip by car, where you spend as many as 10 hours a day with uncomfortable children asking regularly, "Are we there yet?" The stiff back and legs, the hot sun through the glass, the squabbling in the backseat — you wonder why you didn't stay home. But don't do that. Instead, fit in some exercise both in and out of the car to make all of you more manageable.

But enough whining. We need to learn to make the best of modern-day travel because it's all we've got. So buckle up your seat belts, say no to the peanuts, and pay attention. Your course on finding fitness for the road is about to begin.

TOP TEN WAYS TO FIND EXERCISE WHERE THERE IS NONE

The suggestions that follow utilize, once again, that essential muscle for incorporating exercise into your life at home as well as on the road: your imagination.

1. *Learn to think of exercise as any available resistance.* If it has weight, it can be lifted. All phone books, portable televisions, and gaudy lamps qualify.

2. *Remember that when no conventional resistance is available, you can create your own through isometric exercise.* You simply pit your muscles' own powers against themselves.

3. *Bear in mind that most time standing could be spent walking.* You're in a long line at the baggage counter or hotel check-in? Take your luggage for a short hike. Be aware of the time of your flight, of course, but burn calories when you can.

4. *Keep in mind that most time spent sitting could be spent toning and building strength.* Just because your legs can't do much in that straitjacket of an airline seat or the "sinkhole" they call a seat nowadays on trains, that doesn't mean your arms and abs can't be exercised through isometrics.

5. **Learn that most time spent lying down could be spent being far more physically active.** Sleeping is off-limits, of course, but any other time you get a chance to lie down, use that horizontal position to your health's advantage by doing leg lifts, abdominal crunches, even bench presses with weights — or anything else with some gravitational pull. (Great while watching TV aboard beds and couches alike.)

6. **Remember that looking a little odd can be a plus.** If and when you're caught in the act of doing something as absurd-looking as "dips" from the arms of your airplane seat or office chair (see page 95), be honest about what you're up to. Tell any onlooker that you're just trying to get a little exercise in this overly comfortable world. Then offer to demonstrate how those dips are done.

7. **Learn to say no to bellboys.** Politely say thanks but no thanks, tip generously, and be on your way with baggage in hand.

8. **Bear in mind that never, ever should you pass up a flight of stairs.** Remember that step aerobics was invented for a reason.

9. **Learn to be less greedy.** Take your exercise in nickels and dimes rather than waiting for opportunities to get it in large bills. Just a few minutes' worth can be worthwhile.

10. **Remember to be more polite.** Scoff if you like, but the calories burned by such minuscule niceties as holding elevator doors, opening car doors, approaching people rather than shouting to them, and shaking hands more firmly can add up. Besides, you'll probably have more friends.

66 Try to have good walking shoes with you, especially in your car, and always wear them when you travel. That way you can find a way to use waiting time productively. Never pass up the chance to walk. 99

ROB, speech writer

What to Pack for Exercise En Route

Finding fitness on the road can be far easier if you pay attention to what you pack. This doesn't mean emptying out your locker, but it does mean including a few basics.

■ **A Lycra exercise outfit.** Light in weight, Lycra also absorbs very little sweat, meaning it will have a better chance than other materials of drying in time to prevent any unwanted tainting of the rest of your luggage. (This risk can be reduced further by carrying a nylon sport bag with moisture proof compartments designed with this potential hazard in mind.)

■ **Your favorite exercise shoes.** Running shoes, walking shoes, cross-training shoes — it doesn't matter what type they are as long as they're the ones you'll be most likely to use.

■ **Two pairs of socks.** The last thing you want tripping you up on the road is blisters. But just in case they do, also include . . .

■ **Adhesive bandages.** These are especially important if you're breaking in new shoes.

■ **Sunblock.** You don't want the good idea of a midday walk turning into the bad idea of a sunburn.

■ **Athletic "support-wear."** Males, you know what you need; females, the same.

■ **A jump rope.** Jumping rope remains one of the most potent calorie-blasters going, perfect for doing on those plush hotel room carpets.

■ **Elastic exercise "bands."** Not the most engaging devices to use, but a great way to exercise lots of muscle groups in very little space and for very little weight. Several designs are available from several different manufacturers: check your local sporting goods store.

■ **Arm pulleys.** These inexpensive devices are easy to carry and easy to use. Great for toning and strengthening arms and shoulders.

> But isn't all that gear going to make your luggage heavy? All the more to exercise with!

Long plane flights probably are the most discombobulating of all the traveling experiences we face, but they don't have to be. Try some of the following on your next flight, and the skies you fly might not seem so unfriendly after all.

Prevent "dead legs" by getting up from your seat at least every 20 minutes. Walk to the front of the plane or walk to the back of the plane, but be sure to walk. Your goal with these brief treks is not to burn gobs of calories, but rather to prevent excessive pooling of blood in your legs. This circulatory hiatus can be especially uncomfortable if you suffer from varicose veins, but anyone can end up walking like Frankenstein upon landing if preventive measures such as the one above are not taken. Request an aisle seat when booking your flight to make your frequent sojourns less annoying to the person — dead-legged — who is seated next to you.

Work your "buns" with stationary tush-tighteners. Muscles can be exercised without movement. The concept is known as "isometric" exercise and it's a godsend for frequent flyers. To work the muscles of the buttocks using this technique, tighten the muscles of your posterior and hold this flex for about 6 seconds. Relax for several seconds and repeat until you've completed a set of 10. Repeat every half hour or so.

Work your "abs" with upright sit-ups. That's correct, you needn't lie down to work your abdominal muscles (which should make your flight attendant happy). Brace yourself by putting your palms on your thighs just above your knees and attempt to lean forward with slightly bent arms, held rigid. Concentrate on flexing your abs, providing resistance with your arms as you do. You should feel a significant flexing of your abdominal muscles and also a flexing of the triceps (the muscles at the back of your arm), which are providing the resistance. This exercise can be done quite unobtrusively; not even the person seated next to you need know what you're up to. Do sets of 10 every half hour or so, holding each flex for approximately 6 seconds. (Feel free to use this exercise any other time you find yourself needing to be seated for extended periods, such as at your desk; on long car, bus, or train rides; during long-winded presentations; even as a way of getting some ab work during one of those sleep-inducing, epic-length movies.)

Work your biceps with stationary "curls." To use the isometric approach to exercise the muscles of your arms (biceps mainly, but also triceps and forearms), face the palm of your right arm upward and place the palm of your left arm on top of it, facing downward. Now attempt to lift upward with your right arm while using your left arm to prevent you from doing so. You should feel considerable tension in the bicep muscle of your right arm, as well as in the tricep muscle of your left arm. Hold this flex for about 6 seconds, then reverse the procedure to work the bicep of your left arm and tricep of your right. (Refer to the illustration in Appendix A if you're confused.) Repeat this sequence for 10 repetitions, and you'll have gotten an arm workout extraordinaire.

Work your triceps with "dips." The tricep is the major muscle at the back of the arm and can be targeted nicely by pressing up out of your seat using your arms, palms facing down on the armrests at your sides (this also works nicely for office chairs with arms). Try to do a set of 10 every 20 minutes or so (perhaps explaining what you're up to so your seat partner doesn't think you have a problem).

Work your chest muscles with the "prayer." Work your chest muscles ("pecs") in this isometric fashion: Put your palms together in front of your chest (yes, as if saying a prayer) and press together as hard as you can for about 6 seconds. Release for several seconds, then repeat the procedure 10 times. (You'll be getting essentially the same workout as you would by using what's known in health club lingo as a "pec deck," a unit weighing several hundred pounds!)

Diaphragmatic Breathing

Practice this kind of breathing for increased oxygenization — translated, that means increased energy!

1. Place your hands on your ribs under the breast area. Breathe in through your nose, causing your hands to push apart.
2. Breathe out through your mouth. Your hands should come together again.

Try to breathe this way at least once a day for about a week, and eventually it will begin to come naturally.

Work your thighs against the seat ahead of you. The exercises above have worked your abs, arms, chest, and rear — not bad considering you haven't moved from your seat. But to target your legs and make your airline workout complete, try locking your feet beneath the seat in front of you and attempt to lift upward. You'll be working your quadriceps, the large muscles at the front of your thighs, as you do. Make these exertions for about 6 seconds, same as with the exercises above, and again, repeat 10 times.

Work your circulatory system with diaphragmatic breathing. Using your breath to circulate fresh, oxygenated blood through your body will help you feel refreshed and alert.

FITNESS BETWEEN FLIGHTS

Ah, yes. The layover — that uniquely agonizing experience of having to kill time, knowing full well that as soon as you arrive at your destination you'll have to kill *for* it.

So *don't* just kill that time. Put it to use in any number of the following heart-healthy, fat-fighting ways:

Take a hike. If you have one of those killer layovers

(too short to do anything but long enough to bore the pants off you), go for a walk. Find a locker for your baggage and get moving. Indoors, outdoors, it's up to you. Your only restriction: no escalators or moving walkways allowed. Try to keep moving for at least 20 minutes, and don't be afraid to push yourself. You're going to be stuck back on that plane before you know it, so some honest fatigue, if you can achieve it, will feel mighty good.

Secrets of a Super-Fit Salesman

At age 42, Ed is in the best shape of his life. He can do 25 chin-ups, bench press 280 pounds, and play a mean game of tennis and a respectable game of golf. Yet Ed's life ("or at least about two-thirds of it," he estimates) is spent behind the wheel of a very tired Honda. Ed, you see, is the quintessential traveling salesman, his "territory" being the entire southeast quadrant of the United States.

How does he do it?

Looking more like Arnold Schwarzenegger than Willie Loman, Ed was nice enough to reveal his routine:

■ "I do a set of push-ups, abdominal crunches, and about five minutes of running in place before I take a shower and leave my motel room in the morning.

■ "Then, after about three hours of driving, I get off whatever major highway I'm on, find an appropriate area, and go for a 30-minute walk or run, whichever I'm more in the mood for. I carry a spritz bottle of water and paper towels with me in the car so I can clean up afterward as best I can. I'll repeat this in the afternoon, too, if my schedule permits.

■ "When I'm checked back into another motel room at night, I pull out my heavy artillery — my set of dumbbells and portable chin-up bar. If the motel has a pool, I may also go for a swim, or if the area is nice, I'll go for another walk or jog."

Go for a strength walk. This is an alternative to the conventional walk suggested above and is especially suitable for layovers of less than 20 minutes or so. Instead of storing your luggage this time, take it with you. Best of all for strength walks is a balanced load — equally weighted suitcases in either hand — but if you have only one bag, switch hands approximately every minute to give equal opportunities to all muscles involved. If you can, lift your loads higher than their normal carrying position from time to time, to increase the work you're giving your arms.

Check out a fitness facility. Yes, more and more large airports these days (and even some train terminals) are offering fitness centers you can use for a quick workout of nearly any type you want. Many of these centers are full-sized, state-of-the-art gyms with fitness equipment of all types, including saunas, steam rooms, and pools. You might even enjoy the rest of your flight after a workout in one of these!

FITNESS ON WHEELS

Much of our travel, over short distances and long, is by car, bus, and train, and these rides can leave us feeling about as peppy as a mummy. But there are ways to combat that deadening sensation. (Chapters 3 and 4 contain a multitude of exercises that can be done while sitting, and many can be adapted for use in a vehicle. Those and the ones described below can be found in Appendix A.)

When driving: If your trip is more than about an hour, make stops every 45 minutes or so to go for a short walk and do some light stretching. Touch your toes, swing your arms in large circles, roll your head from side to side to loosen your neck. Not only will you feel better when you return to the wheel, you'll be more alert.

When riding: Whether in a car, train, or bus, riding can be even more "stiffening" than driving because you don't even have the steering wheel and pedals to occupy your hands and feet. So give them something else to do!

- Do Isometric Curls (page 146) for your arms to wake up your upper body.

- Do upright sit-ups (page 94) for your abdomen.

- Do Shoulder Rolls and Shoulder Shrugs (pages 159, 160) to relieve tension in your shoulders and neck.

- Squeeze a small rubber ball or a tennis ball to work the muscles of the forearms and wrists. (Squeeze it when you feel like squeezing the necks of some of your fellow passengers, perhaps.)

- If you're aboard a train or bus, don't be shy about getting up and walking to the rest room (even if you don't need to). A short sojourn every 10 minutes or so can do wonders at maintaining adequate blood flow to the legs.

HOW TO RUN TWO MILES IN A HOTEL ROOM

If your hotel has a fitness facility, do your body, brain, and boss (assuming your company will foot the bill for your travel) the favor of using it. You'll feel better, perform better, even look better.

But what if your lodging does *not* have such a facility?

Devise a workout you can do in your room, one that not only will relieve stress but also will burn calories and give a strength workout, too.

If you've put together an indoor morning exercise routine (as discussed in chapter 3), chances are you can do it in your hotel room just as easily, as long as you don't rely on extra equipment that doesn't fit in a suitcase. Or you can sweat along with a TV aerobics show before stepping into the shower.

That's right. Scenic it's not, but fast and effective it most certainly is. In just 15 minutes, you can burn approximately 200 calories if you put your heart into it. And a good workout may help you to sleep better in this less-than-homey environment.

The 15-Minute-Anywhere Workout

Upon returning home from the two-week trip that inspired me to devise this workout, I ran the speediest marathon of my life. Was it because the workout merely had given me rest from my normal, more grueling routine? Perhaps, but even so, it certainly did a good job.

 ### The Cardiovascular Portion

- 3 minutes of jumping jacks
- 3 minutes of running in place
- 3 minutes of jumping rope

 ### The Strength-Building Portion

- 1 set of Arm Circles* or push-ups (if you've already developed the necessary arm strength, do as many as you can)
- 1 set of Isometric Curls*
- 1 set of Semi Sit-Ups*

 ### The Flexibility Portion

- 5–10 Jackknife stretches*
- 5–10 Hip and Thigh Stretchers*

See Appendix A

Fitness Through Sports

M ike used to jog. And when he was jogging, he would sometimes pass people playing softball, tennis, or golf, or someone throwing a Frisbee to a dog. Mike would chuckle to himself as he'd watch these "exercise impostors," as he called them — people who were moving around but for naught, because their activities were neither strenuous enough nor sustained for a long enough period to do them any appreciable good.

Mike was a die-hard "target-heart-rate" guy, you see, a committed follower of aerobic doctrine in its purest form. He would go so far as to run in place at stop lights during his jogs, afraid that his precious heart rate might fall below its fitness-producing target zone if he stood still for even a few seconds.

Needless to say, Mike didn't enjoy running. He despised it, in fact, but he was convinced that unless he *did* despise it, it probably wasn't doing him any good. The "no-pain, no-gain" credo had carved out a permanent niche in his brain. Maybe you know Mike's type. Maybe you *are* Mike's type.

If so, our condolences, because in addition to missing the point about exercise, you're missing out on ways to improve

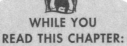

**WHILE YOU
READ THIS CHAPTER:**
Sit with knees together. Move knees to the
left while moving head and neck to the right, keeping chin
tucked and feet flat on floor. Repeat, alternating sides, for a total of 10.

your fitness that could be a lot of fun. Yes, research leaves no doubt that running remains one of the most time-efficient activities for burning calories and building cardiovascular endurance, but that doesn't automatically make it the best path to fitness for everyone. There's the all-important "is-it-likely-to-be-done" factor to consider, plus the risk of injury. In light of that, running for many people is *not* such an ideal exercise — die-hard Mike, unfortunately, being the proof.

Scoff as he might at the softball players and Frisbee throwers, Mike eventually aggravated a ligament in his knee, refused to stop running despite his doctor's advice, and now, 20 pounds heavier, has trouble even walking for fitness.

THE RUN VS. THE HOME RUN

Time out, you say? You think that running and other hard-core aerobic activities may have their drawbacks, but there's no way that spending the better part of a Saturday afternoon getting bitten by mosquitoes in right field is going to get you fit, much less burn enough calories to help you control your weight? You think you'd be better off going for a 30-minute jog, even if it's once in a blue moon?

Not so fast. Some quick arithmetic will show that's not necessarily true. Two hours of playing softball (providing they're not spent mostly eating hot dogs and drinking beer) can burn approximately 500 calories for someone who weighs 150 pounds. Pitchers and catchers can burn even more — as many as 750 calories in two hours if their hearts are really in the game.

Compare these figures to the calories burned by a 30-minute jog at a 10-minute-per-mile pace — about 300 — and you can see that the game of softball is not such a day at the beach after all. Other sports burn substantially more calories than does softball (see chart on page 107), so there definitely are some health benefits to be gained just for the fun of it.

Don't get me wrong. Aerobic exercise in its traditional forms of running, cycling, swimming, and the like is a tremendous way to burn calories and great for strengthening the cardiovascular system. But less arduous endeavors, such as a good softball or touch football game, can also be worthy fitness efforts.

LET COMPETITION DEFEAT YOUR FAT

Team sports are good for you and enjoyable, too, and yet so seemingly *easy*, which may be the greatest fitness advantage these activities have. Even though the movements they require can be quite demanding, the effort expended in performing them sometimes seems mystifyingly easy, given the spirit of competition in which they're made. Streak for home plate en route to scoring your team's winning run, for example, or run hard for a winning shot in a game of tennis, and the last thing you're thinking about is your heart rate or the number of calories you're burning. You're thinking about the *game*.

Even if you aren't sliding headfirst into home plate or outlasting your opponent in a marathon game of tennis, you're still burning more calories than you would by watching these sports on TV. Remember, the latest research shows that any activity, regardless of its intensity or duration, is immensely better than no activity at all, especially for people not accustomed to much physical exertion. The

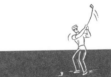

❝ I love team sports for exercise because the excitement of the game and competition make it fun. Most of the time I forget that I'm also exercising. When I'm chasing someone down, rounding the bases, or driving to the hoop, I'm concentrating on the game, not on exercising. **❞**

NANCY, recent college graduate

> *"The best exercise for anybody is the exercise
> they're most likely to do."*
>
> Dr. Bryant Stamford

very fact that you're at least *out there* on the softball field or basketball court instead of glued to the TV is a major point in your favor. It's certainly going to bring you closer to fitness than will staring at a pair of running shoes you can't bear to use or at an exercise contraption that looks like a medieval torture device. As University of Louisville exercise physiologist Dr. Bryant Stamford says, "The best exercise for anybody is the exercise they're most likely to do."

Keep that in mind as you're trying to map out the wisest path to your fitness goals. If you're at all competitive, put that trait to work for your health. *Movement,* not pain, is what expends energy. And fun can be a great fitness ally. When the going gets tough, the tough may get going — but the smart find a more enjoyable way. Consider the following case histories that illustrate this point.

"Losing" by Winning: Carol's Story

Carol, a 42-year-old mother of three, had failed at more weight-loss programs than she could recall, and had lost a lot of self-respect as well as money along the way. Then one day a coworker asked her to try out for the company volleyball team. Her first thought, understandably, was that it was out of the question. At 5 feet 4 inches and 165 pounds, she was certainly no Gabrielle Reece. But her friend wouldn't take no for an answer, so Carol gave it a try.

A phenomenally successful try, as it turns out. Carol discovered something about herself: She had one *heck* of a competitive side. Athletically gifted she was not, but someone who loved to win? Her teammates thought so: They eventually elected her captain of the team. What she lacked in talent she made up for in intensity. Winning gave her ego just the nourishment it so badly needed. It also gave her body the exercise *it* so badly needed.

Within a month of joining the team, Carol had lost almost 10 pounds, and as of this writing she's still going strong. "I haven't really even been trying to lose weight, which is why it's been surprising," she says. "Our games and practices are in the evenings, so I'm careful to eat a light dinner so I don't get nauseated. Then at night I'm usually so pumped up, especially if we've won, that I kind of forget about food. In the old days, food is all I could think about at night."

Carol's new found athleticism also has given her noticeably more energy in everything else she does, which she feels is instrumental in helping her lose weight. "I'm just so much more active now," she says. "My husband and I have rejoined the bowling league we belonged to years ago, and I also do a lot more things on weekends with the kids. Even on evenings when I'm not playing volleyball, I'm more active. I do more around the house and have even started a garden for the first time in about 20 years." And all thanks to the "firing up" of her competitive spirit.

The Challenge of Fitness: Robert's Story

Robert, a 52-year-old executive with a major advertising firm, tells a similar tale.

He had been on the varsity tennis team in college, and while not a star, Robert was no slouch, either. He was an under-achiever, by his own assessment, definitely talented but more interested during that hormonal period of his life in co-eds. Upon graduation, like many college athletes, Robert went into a *long* hibernation — "about 30 years," he says, which coincidentally was good for a weight gain of approximately the same number of pounds.

Then late one night at a cocktail party, Robert was offered a challenge from a younger member of his staff who knew of his boss's former renown: one set, for $1,000, with one month to prepare.

Robert became a man obsessed. Not because of the money: He had earmarked that for charity the night the wager was made. Robert's pride was on the line, and he wasn't going to let it go without a battle. Five nights a week he hit balls against a backboard at the indoor facility of the local country club, and on weekends he enlisted the opposition of his youngest daughter, who was a star player on her high-school team. The night before the showdown, Robert even went to bed without his customary nightcap(s), for the first time in over 20 years.

Space limitations do not permit a blow-by-blow account of Robert's heroic struggle, but suffice it to say that he won by a gallantly contested 7–5 score. More importantly, however, Robert has been banging around that fuzzy little white ball ever since. He competes for his country club and helps to coach his daughter's team, and both his weight and his blood pressure have been on a steady downward path. He has even made a point of breaking his habit of nightly nightcaps.

YOU, TOO, CAN BE A CHAMP

Inspired? Covered with goose bumps? Interested in kicking a little you-know-what yourself?

Good, because sports have been in the aerobic doghouse too long. They provide exercise. They can help with weight loss. They can be a source of fun. And they can be a great source of camaraderie, no matter what the score.

Participating in leisure-time activities that involve physical activity reduces stress, increases enjoyment of life, and builds solid friendships. But it can be even more beneficial to your body — and give you a real sense of victory when you step on the scale.

ACTIVITY	CALORIES BURNED PER HOUR*
Archery	195
Badminton	390
Bowling	175
Croquet	195
Fishing (fly)	195
Golf (carrying bags)	375
Horseback riding (trot)	430
Horseshoes	180
Hunting (small game)	250
In-line skating	400
Racquetball	630
Scuba diving	580
Skiing (cross-country)	580
Skiing (downhill)	400
Soccer	570
Softball	250
Squash	660
Swimming (crawl)	540
Table tennis	300
Tennis (doubles)	270
Tennis (singles)	435
Touch football	420
Volleyball	340
Water skiing	465

(by someone weighing 150 lbs.)

And If All Else Fails, Just Take a Hike

Perhaps the greatest irony of all about our current exercise deficit is how avoidable it's actually been. Yes, technology took the exercise out of our jobs and domestic duties, and we got some overly ambitious advice from our fitness forefathers on how to get that exercise back. But all along a solution has been as close as the soles of our feet. Despite the maze of more elaborate and exhausting options, the road to fitness can be as easily traveled as putting one foot in front of the other. No special equipment needed, no athletic talent — not even a shower because there's no need to break a sweat.

"All things considered, walking is the single most practical and effective form of exercise available to the average American today," says Mark Bricklin, founder of the Prevention Walking Club and the editor of *Prevention* magazine. "No other activity bestows the blessings of exercise as easily, enjoyably, or safely as the simple act of going for a walk."

Evidence supporting Bricklin's claims is impressive. Research shows that compared to exercisers who pursue fitness in other ways, walkers suffer the fewest injuries, have the lowest dropout rate, and continue their programs well into their twilight years.

WHILE YOU READ THIS CHAPTER:
Take a 5-minute, fast-paced walk when you are midway through this chapter and another when you are at the end.

NOT FOR WIMPS ONLY

No surprise, you say, because walking is so "wimpy"? If you could be convinced that it would really do some measurable good, you might give it a go?

Then get ready to lace up, because walking is finally getting the recognition as real exercise that it deserves. And as for walking being for wimps only, you might want to run that one by Texas A&M University anthropologist Vaughn Bryant, who has lots of stories to tell regarding walking's impact on those who first put it to use: our prehistoric ancestors. Walking has been the primary fitness activity of our species ever since we got up off all fours an estimated 1.5 million years ago, Dr. Bryant says. There were no stationary bikes or step-aerobics classes for our fur-clad forebears yet they were extraordinarily fit thanks primarily to their ambulatory ways.

"We were working at a site in Texas, doing exploratory digging in caves set on the side of a canyon wall where a prehistoric tribe had lived," Dr. Bryant says. "And talk about a climb! Of the nineteen of us on the expedition, twelve couldn't make it up the incline even once. Here was something our prehistoric ancestors were doing every day, as routinely as taking out the garbage, and twelve modern young people — college students, no less — couldn't manage it even once."

THE "FOREST" WITHOUT THE "TREES"

Okay, so that's what a life of running from saber-toothed tigers can do?

No, that's what a life of walking can do. "We estimate that on an average hunt, a prehistoric man might have walked about ten miles, and the women and children, whose job it was to gather most of the plant foods, probably walked between four and six miles a day," Dr. Bryant says. "The men might have run at certain times during their hunts, but primarily these ventures were exercises in tracking, so running would have been unlikely." As for the women and children, "they were gathering things, remember, so running would have been even less appropriate for them."

Inappropriate. If that's what running, weight lifting, or any other more frenetic approach to exercise has been for you, take solace from the caveman's tale. He walked his way to fitness, as did his family — just as you and your family can, too. It's easy but also highly effective, it requires no special equipment or athletic ability, and you can do it nearly any time or anywhere without risk of injury or undue fatigue.

Walking can be the "forest," in other words, for all of us whose fitness efforts may have been tripped up by the "trees." It can even *get* us places, and by burning *calories* instead of gas!

"MAN'S BEST MEDICINE" — ESPECIALLY FOR WEIGHT LOSS

If you've yet to find a fitness activity you can live with, walking could be it. Many people take up walking underestimating the positive changes it can make, but soon become hooked when they realize how easy, satisfying, and fat-blasting it can be. In one study done at the University of California (Irvine) Medical Center, a group of obese patients who had repeatedly failed to lose weight by dieting lost an average of 22 pounds when put on a 30-minute-a-day walking program for a year. These losses occurred even though the people made no changes in what they ate.

"The key with walking seems to be that it's one of the few activities people will do with the degree of regularity that effective long-term weight loss requires," says Bricklin. True, jogging burns slightly more calories than walking on a per-mile basis, but when you consider how you feel after a jog as compared to a walk of similar length, you can begin to see why walking takes the weight-loss lead. People invariably exercise more frequently *and* for longer periods of time when they walk instead of jog, and that translates into more calories burned.

Why Walk?

The list of walking's benefits is as irrefutable as it is impressive. Research has found all of the following to be among the reasons you should seriously consider walking as a fitness staple. Just 30 minutes a day, divided any way you choose, is all that's required:

- Improves efficiency of the heart and lungs
- Burns body fat
- Raises metabolism, thus increasing calorie-burning even at rest
- Helps control appetite
- Increases energy
- Helps relieve stress
- Retards aging
- Reduces levels of cholesterol in the blood
- Lowers high blood pressure
- Helps control and prevent adult-onset diabetes
- Reduces risks of some forms of cancer (colorectal, prostate, and breast)
- Aids rehabilitation from heart attack and stroke
- Promotes intestinal regularity
- Helps promote more restful sleep
- Strengthens muscles of the legs, hips, and torso
- Strengthens bones
- Reduces stiffness in joints due to inactivity or arthritis
- Relieves most cases of chronic backache
- Improves flexibility
- Improves posture
- Promotes healthier skin due to increased circulation
- Improves mental alertness and memory
- Spurs intellectual creativity and problem solving
- Elevates mood
- Helps prevent and/or reduce depression
- Improves self-esteem
- Increases sexual vigor
- Helps control addictions to nicotine, alcohol, caffeine, and other drugs

You do get what you "weigh" for with walking, as with all weight-bearing exercise. Walking one mile burns the following number of calories for the body weights given.

BODYWEIGHT	CALORIES BURNED PER MILE
120	80
130	85
140	95
150	100
160	105
170	110
180	115
190	120
200	125

Or as cardiologist James Rippe, of the University of Massachusetts Medical Center, says, "Weight loss truly is a race won by the tortoise rather than the hare."

HOW TO WALK

Even a tortoise has got to get its rear in gear, however, so here are some basic steps for doing so.

Be patient. Some fitness experts say that for every year of inactivity, a month of exercise is needed to make up for it, so gauge your efforts accordingly. By pushing yourself too hard, you risk forcing your body to rebel in the form of soreness, injury, or undue fatigue. Your goal should be to build up to at least 30 minutes of walking a day, but feel free to take at least a month to do that if your current fitness level is low.

Put consistency ahead of intensity or speed. Better to walk a little every day than to go long distances with frequent days off: You give your body a better idea of the changes you're trying to make.

Breathe with fitness in mind. Breathe rhythmically and deeply as you walk (but not so deeply that you could not comfortably converse with someone: You'll risk having to cut your walks short if you do).

Add some stretching to your walking program. Failure to do so can lead to tightness in the muscles of the hamstrings, located at the rear of the upper thighs, and the muscles of the lower back. (See Appendix A for stretching ideas.)

Get yourself some decent shoes. Shoes designed specifically for walking are best, so put your money where your feet are.

Pay attention to form. That can sound silly given that you've been walking for quite some time now, but proper form is important. You'll achieve more fitness, suffer less soreness, and have more fun. (See below.)

The Way to Walk

Proper form can make all the difference between an energizing and enjoyable walk (one you'll be eager to repeat) and an exhausting ordeal. Follow these tips to make sure your walk will be an experience you'll look forward to rather than dread.

- Walk with your back straight and head held erect, your toes pointed straight ahead and your arms swinging at your sides at approximately a 90° angle.

- Land on your heels and roll forward to drive off the balls of your feet. Walking flat-footed can cause soreness and premature fatigue.

- Lean slightly forward and pump harder with your arms when going uphill.

- To walk faster, increase your cadence rather than the length of your stride, which can risk injury to the knees.

The data on walking is in: It's a sure winner, and one that more and more of us are coming around to as an ideal fitness activity. Here are some interesting facts on our oldest form of exercise that may help increase your motivation.

- Walking within 30 minutes after eating can boost calorie-burning by as much as 30 percent.
- Walking in sand, loose soil, or deep grass also can increase calorie-burning by as much as 30 percent.
- Walking up hills can increase calorie-burning by as much as 45 percent.
- The energy costs of walking can be increased by 78 percent by walking backward (recommended for open spaces only).
- Walking a mile in 15 minutes burns as many calories as running a mile in 8½ minutes.
- Walking a mile a day (in addition to your usual activity) could result in a fat loss of approximately one pound per month.
- A quality treadmill can give an exceptionally good walking workout (and even more convenience) by ensuring a steady pace.
- Walkers currently outnumber runners 5 to 1.
- Walking is the fastest growing fitness activity in America today.
- Walking at a 4–5 MPH pace (approximately 15 minutes per mile) burns as many calories as belly dancing.
- The foot might seem simple enough, but it has 26 separate bones, 30 different muscles, 56 tendons, 250,000 sweat glands, and 33 joints.
- Myth: Walking barefoot can flatten the feet (it simply thickens the skin on the bottoms of the feet).
- Walking can help the body with its sizable chore of producing new bone tissue — the equivalent of a whole new skeleton every seven years.
- Walking in high heels can subject the ball of the foot to as many as 2,000 pounds of pressure with every step.
- Think acrylic when thinking socks: They stay drier, fit better, and dry faster than cotton.
- To help loosen a knotted shoelace, sprinkle it with talc.
- Best anthropological reason to take up walking: It most closely re-creates the exercise conditions under which our bodies evolved.

A word about hand-held weights. Studies show that calorie-burning is *not* increased appreciably by walking with weights, although the practice can help tone the muscles of the arms. Hold weights — 2 to 3 pounds but no more than 5 — with arms bent and swinging normally. (Ankle weights are *not* recommended because they can increase risk of injury by altering foot placement and stride.)

STEPS TO A HIGHER I.Q.?

Despite being such a simple activity, walking has earned some contemplative followers. Wordsworth relied on walking for his greatest insights, averaging 14 miles a day and once hiking 350 miles through Europe to aid his poetic muse. Thoreau also was an avid ambler (reportedly covering 250,000 miles in his lifetime), as were Benjamin Franklin, Thomas Jefferson, Abraham Lincoln, and Albert Einstein. The noted existentialist and dedicated perambulator Nietzsche went so far as to contend that "only those thoughts that come by walking have any value."

As poorly as that notion may sit with the legion of armchair philosophers around the world, it does make a valid point regarding walking's stimulating effects on the mind. The degree of exertion required by walking seems to be perfect for infusing the brain with the right amounts of glucose and oxygen for optimal enhancement of the thought process. Add the soothing rhythm of the walking stride and it's no wonder so many of the world's greatest thinkers did their best brainstorming afoot — as you can, too.

To Equip or Not to Equip

There are two opposing schools of thought among exercisers regarding the use of equipment in the pursuit of fitness. One is the purist view, which sees exercise equipment as a pathetic excuse for the real thing, best suited for wimps and dreamers more likely to derive satisfaction from owning the stuff than from actually using it. These people can be found "just doing it" regardless of weather conditions or sometimes even in the dark of night.

The other school is less fanatic. It maintains that exercise equipment is a logical extension of the progress that took the "real thing" away from us in the first place. Those who share this belief readily avail themselves of gadgetry that can range from the ingenious to the absurd.

Which view is closer to the truth?

They both miss the point. The exercise that's right is the exercise that's right for *you*, whether it's riding a runner's high, a stationary bike, a horse, or a wave. What's important is the degree of connection you have with the activity. It must be something you're likely to repeat, whether in pursuit of another trophy or just a flatter stomach.

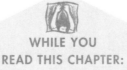

**WHILE YOU
READ THIS CHAPTER:**
Slowly raise your shoulders toward your ears.
Hold for 10 seconds and release. Repeat 3 times.

But then, if too much of the "real thing" leads to injury, you might have no *choice* but to turn to one of those gizmos. Real exercise is great if you can get it, and stand up to it, but for the millions of us not so fortunate or so durable, exercise equipment can be a lifesaver.

BE SURE THE METAL HAS METTLE

Before falling for the next gut-buster, hip-chiseler, or thigh-slasher you see, know that there are the good, the bad, and the ugly in this ever-expanding market of exercise gear. Some stuff is highly effective, brilliantly designed, engaging to use, and amazingly sturdy.

Other devices, however, are engineering embarrassments, designed with the full expectation that they will collect more dust than sweat. To help you distinguish the gems from the junk, here are some shopping strategies:

1. *Decide on your fitness goals.* This might sound obvious, but with the warehouse of stuff that's out there, you can get lost if you don't. If your primary goal is to burn calories for weight control, look at devices capable of giving you a good cardiovascular workout. Those include treadmills, stationary bikes, stair-climbing machines, cross-country skiers, and rowing machines.

If toning and strengthening muscles are your main interests, however, a device designed to offer resistance is a better choice. Many multiexercise weight machines are now available for this purpose, as are good old-fashioned barbells, dumbbells, and, most recently, a whole new family of tubing and bands capable of providing good strength-building struggles. Highly portable, these recent additions can be good choices if you'd like the option of taking your muscle-toning with you on the road.

2. *Don't buy until you try.* This advice comes from the High Technology Fitness Institute and can, indeed, save you headaches as well as money. As convincing as those infomercials can be, there's nothing like a real "test drive" to see if a given gadget is going to suit you in both fit and feel. But what can you do if the unit you want is being sold on TV only, or through a catalog?

Then look for the device or one similar to it in a department or sporting goods store, or hunt one down at a health club, or find a friend who has one. Do your very best not to buy any equipment without trying it, no matter how convincing its ex-Olympic spokesperson may sound.

3. *Shop at a reputable store (or do some intelligent comparison shopping).* Many of the above uncertainties can be minimized by shopping at a reputable fitness equipment outlet. You might pay a little more, but given the dangers of buying based on celebrity value alone, it can be well worth it. Explain to the salesperson your fitness goals, how often you plan to use the device, whether anyone else will be using it, and where you're hoping to put the unit in your home. Some equipment — weight machines and treadmills especially — can be heavy enough to pose a real threat of doing serious structural damage if installed where support is not adequate, so be sure to consult your salesperson before attempting anything that may be architecturally risky.

It Takes Two

What type of exercise equipment is best? Most experts agree that it's probably best to get two: a cardiovascular trainer *plus* a means of improving muscular tone and strength. Variety is the spice of fitness as well as life, after all, so why *not* a device for burning calories and strengthening the heart one day, and a way to tone and shape muscles the next? You'll reduce your chances of injury due to overuse this way, and you'll also be mounting a two-pronged attack in your war against weight gain: a cardiovascular activity for burning calories as you're actually doing it, plus a strength-building workout for giving your muscles the pizzazz they need to be better calorie-burners even when they're just helping you watch TV.

If you already know what you want and why you want it, however, by all means shop the classifieds. There are as many great deals out there as there are, sadly, people still in the dark about how to find a lasting relationship with exercise.

4. Let quality and comfort be your guides. What should you look for once aboard a potential purchase?

First of all, stability. There should be no rock, rattle, or roll. Beware, too, of an overuse of plastic, which can fatigue with heavy use even before you do. After that, it's all about comfort. Pay attention to how the unit actually feels. Does it cause you pain anywhere when you use it? Is the level of exertion it requires too intense, or not intense enough? Can you see yourself using it — without dread or despair — on a consistent basis for the rest of your life?

If not, keep shopping.

5. Think twice about the bells and whistles. Do you really need the computer screen that lets you cycle the Swiss Alps? Or the heart-rate monitor that's going to be giving you a virtual EKG?

If so, fine, but don't be talked into such high-tech gadgetry because you fear your fitness will suffer if you just say no. Such extras jack up not only the price of what you buy, but also the potential for breakdown and subsequent need for repairs. Also be savvy about your unit's warranty; it should be good for at least 90 days and cover both parts and service.

6. Determine whether you'll be able to do something else while you work out. Some devices are better than others for allowing you to read while you exercise — stationary bikes, steppers, and treadmills, for example, are more suitable than rowers and cross-country skiers, where the head remains less consistently in a stable position. With the first group of devices you'll be able to make or take phone calls, if that's important to you, because they involve less activity with the arms and hands. Just about all exercise equipment, however, can be used while listening to music, books on tape, or self-help material through headphones, or as you watch TV or movies on a VCR, which can help pass the time.

LOOK BEFORE YOU LEAP INTO A HEALTH CLUB

But why buy, when for a nominal monthly fee you can join a gym or health club that has an exercise machine for every muscle of your body, not to mention full-length mirrors and instructors that look like they came off the set of *Baywatch*?

Careful. There's the all-important inconvenience factor to consider, one that keeps two out of three health club members from using a facility more than 100 days a year, according to research by American Sports Data. Surveys also show that two out of three club members work out at home about 50 percent as often as they do at their clubs, so the experience, while seemingly ideal, obviously has its drawbacks.

This is not meant to bury health clubs; they warrant praise, but with some provisos. If you're someone who likes structure and would welcome some hands-on instruction and wouldn't mind an occasional wait for the likes of the "pec-deck" and wouldn't be intimidated by a lot of Arnold Schwarzenegger and Pamela Lee look-alikes, then go for it. Do consider the extra time it's going to take to get there, however, and that you may have to dress a little differently from the way you do at home.

But if it's the chrome, the smell of sweat, and the full-length mirrors you want, a health club is the place. To keep from losing your shirt along with whatever pounds you may drop, however, do some investigation before signing any contracts. Here are the key questions to ask.

What do I get for my membership? Most clubs offer a free fitness evaluation plus a session with an instructor to set up a program designed specifically for you.

Can I sell my membership to someone else? If you should decide you want out of your membership, your club may permit you to sell the remainder. Don't assume this is the case, though. Check it out before you sign up.

Can I get a refund if I'm injured or have to move? Some clubs limit refunds, and some clubs refuse them altogether.

Can I get a discount for using the club at odd hours? Daytime weekday rates should be lower if your club offers this feature.

Can I use facilities in other cities if the club is part of a chain? This is important to know if you travel a lot.

What qualifications and training do the instructors have? Check with the American Council on Exercise (800-529-8227) to learn what to look for.

Is the club's equipment leased or owned? Leasing is preferable because the equipment is apt to be more up-to-date.

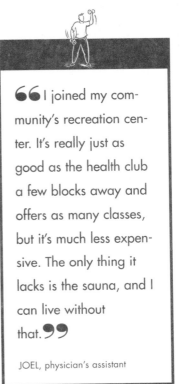

66 I joined my community's recreation center. It's really just as good as the health club a few blocks away and offers as many classes, but it's much less expensive. The only thing it lacks is the sauna, and I can live without that. **99**

JOEL, physician's assistant

Will I have to wait for extended periods to use any of the machines? Try to drop in during peak hours to see what machines are in use.

Are there hours when parts of the facility are off-limits because of special classes or workouts for local teams? Pools are often reserved for this purpose.

Will the club let me have my own copy of the contract? If not, take your body elsewhere.

Will the club demand a down payment before I've had a chance to read the contract? If so, definitely go elsewhere.

Last but not least, talk to some of the club's clients and get their impressions. If they're not happy, odds are you won't be, either.

If you can't afford health clubs but yearn for their structure, check out cheaper alternatives such as your local Y, Jewish Community Center, or college exercise facilities.

THE SKINNY ON PERSONAL TRAINERS

Are they for celebrities and company presidents only?

Not necessarily, says the American Association for Physical Fitness Education. If expense is no obstacle and the hand-holding is something you honestly think might help you, or you have an illness or disability that makes it difficult for you to exercise on your own — by all means, give a personal trainer (PT) a shot.

Do not, however, enlist the services of any well-tanned hunk who might come banging on your door. Here are three things to look for in a PT, says the American Association for Physical Fitness Education:

- **Certification by the American Council on Exercise.** There are now 13,000 ACE-certified personal trainers worldwide, up from 2,000 since 1990.
- **Affiliation with a fitness center, health club, or YWCA or YMCA.** Reputable organizations always screen their associates.
- **References from satisfied clients.**

Ask other clients about the trainer's ability to design a well-rounded fitness program that includes not just cardiovascular work but also strength training and muscle toning, stretching exercises, dietary advice, posture assessment, and breathing and relaxation techniques.

The fee you can expect to pay for such a gym bag of services?

Between $25 and $75 an hour, depending on where you live and the experience and reputation of the person you're hiring. Anything more, and the *trainer* had better be a celebrity.

For information on how to find a reliable personal trainer in your area, call the American Council on Exercise (800-529-8227).

The Difference Diet Can Make

I n light of the latest research and what the Surgeon General's Report on Physical Activity and Health has to say, no one will deny that exercise is of utmost importance to our health, and more so now than ever before.

But we need more than exercise to get fit. No amount of activity can make as much as a dent in a love handle if we don't also watch what we eat. Yes, exercise can burn the calories it takes to lose weight, but not if more of those calories are coming in than the exercise is burning. And, yes, exercise can help protect you from heart disease and a slew of other major illnesses, but not if it's being fueled by a diet too high in fat.

Diet, you see, has the power to be the great eraser: All the good that exercise can do, diet can undo even better.

But eating healthfully is too complicated, you say? You can't see yourself counting grams much less milligrams?

Relax. Despite the avalanche of allegedly "new" health information that overwhelms us in magazines and diet books, the quieter understanding within the scientific community is that healthful eating can be far simpler than the stampede of magazine articles and diet books would have us believe. The body's chemistry is essentially the same as it's been for the past

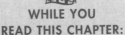

**WHILE YOU
READ THIS CHAPTER:**
Place your palms together in front of your chest.
Press your hands together as hard as you can for 5 seconds.
Repeat for a total of 5 times.

250 million years, you see. The diet we need is simply one that contains more of the basic food on which we evolved.

But before we get into just what that food is, let's find out how badly you need it. Perhaps you've got your Ph.D. in healthful eating already. But then again, maybe you're still at the kindergarten level, in which case you'll need to learn the basic ground ABCs of good nutrition.

Take the following test to find out just how healthful your diet is.

How Healthful Is Your Diet?

To tally your score, give yourself one point for every "A" answer, two for every "B," three for each "C," and four for every "D." See the remarks at the end of the quiz to find out what your score portends.

1. My usual eating pattern is:
  A. to kind of graze all day long
  B. to sit down to three fairly traditional "squares"
  C. to skip breakfast or lunch
  D. to skip breakfast and lunch

2. My usual number of servings of vegetables a day is:
  A. three or more
  B. two
  C. one
  D. zero

3. The breakfast that most closely resembles my usual one is:
  A. a high-vitamin cereal with low-fat milk and some juice or fresh fruit
  B. toast or a bagel with butter and jam, along with juice or fresh fruit
  C. eggs, bacon or sausage, and toast
  D. a Danish or doughnut, or no breakfast at all

4. When at a restaurant, and the potatoes offered are baked, mashed, or french fried, I usually order:

A. baked potato

2← B. mashed potatoes

C. french fries

D. french fries with melted cheese

5. Most of the protein in my diet comes from:

1← A. chicken, turkey, or fish, usually baked or broiled

B. beef and pork

C. cheese and other dairy products such as cream cheese and milk

D. fast-food entrées such as Whoppers and Big Macs

6. If I'm hungry and there's nothing but a vending machine around, I'll have:

A. a piece of fresh fruit if it's available, or nothing at all

B. a package of dry-roasted nuts

3← C. a pack of peanut butter or cheese crackers

D. a candy bar

7. My usual salad dressing is:

A. a good wine or balsamic vinegar

2← B. one of the new low-fat or nonfat dressings

C. oil and vinegar

D. Russian, Roquefort, French, Italian, or blue cheese

8. When I eat at a fast-food restaurant, I usually order:

A. I try not to eat at fast-food restaurants

B. low-fat items from the salad bar

3— C. a low-fat entrée such as a broiled chicken sandwich, plain flame-broiled burger, or a bowl of chili

D. the tallest, cheesiest, sauciest sandwich on the menu, preferably topped with bacon

9. The milk I usually use on my cereal and/or in my coffee is:

A. skim

B. 1% fat

3— C. 2% fat

D. regular

10. When at a party, the hors d'oeuvres I usually eat are:
A. raw vegetables, such as carrot sticks, celery, and broccoli and cauliflower florets
B. cheese and crackers
C. Swedish meatballs
D. little hot dogs and/or deep-fried cheese balls

11. The butter or margarine in my diet comes mostly from:
A. I try not to use butter or margarine
B. the small amount I use in cooking
C. the moderate amount I use on my toast for breakfast and maybe baked or mashed potatoes for dinner
D. the copious amounts I put on nearly anything that will hold it: pancakes, sandwiches, potatoes, vegetables, and especially my extra-large bucket of oil-popped popcorn at the movies

12. The refined white sugar in my diet comes mostly from:
A. the little bit that might be in the few processed foods I eat
B. the little bit I add to my coffee
C. whatever may be in the candy bars, sodas, and desserts I sometimes eat
D. what I put on my cereal and in my coffee, plus whatever may be in the candy bars, sodas, desserts, and bonbons I snack on almost nightly

13. My most frequently consumed snack foods are:
A. air-popped popcorn (without butter) and rice cakes
B. pretzels, preferably unsalted
C. chips — potato or corn
D. pork rinds, beef jerky, and pig's knuckles

14. The last time I had a packaged pastry product such as a Twinkie was:
A. when I was in grade school
B. when I was in high school
C. when I was trying to live on $10 a week in college
D. I am having a Twinkie right now

SCORING

12 — 20: High honors. Congratulations. Your diet is giving your body every advantage it deserves.

21 — 27: Honorable mention. Nice going. Your diet is certainly better than most, but still could use some improvement.

28 — 33: Meritorious. Your diet could be worse, but it also could be far better, as could your energy level and health.

34 — 39: UN-meritorious. Your diet is approaching abominable, and it's only a matter of time until your body begins to pay a price. Please pay close attention to the nutritional advice that follows.

40 and beyond: DIS-honorable mention. Your diet is thwarting your health with every bite. Please pay especially close attention to the nutritional advice that follows.

10 COMMANDMENTS FOR EATING FOR THE HEALTH OF IT

We may not be exactly what we eat, but we come pretty close. Research suggests that as much as 75 percent of all illnesses we suffer in the United States may be in some way diet-related, and this goes for fatal and nonfatal maladies alike. Whether it's heart disease, cancer, stroke, diabetes, high blood pressure, osteoporosis, or arthritis — or just general fatigue and a tendency to catch every cold and flu that comes down the pike — diet is usually involved. So what better reason to tidy up your table manners than that? Especially if you are, in fact, so super-busy? You don't have *time* to get sick.

What follows are the top 10 dietary rules as generally agreed upon by the American Heart Association, the

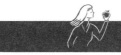

66 Before I took up running, I never paid much attention to my diet. Running has made me more aware of how my body performs. I can see a big difference for the worse when I've eaten fatty foods or not enough protein. 99

MARK, social worker

American Cancer Society, the National Cancer Institute, the Center for Science in the Public Interest, the American Council on Exercise, and many independent nutritionists.

Before you stop reading right here, assuming that any dietary recommendations coming from these organizations has got to be pretty depressing, know that just the opposite can be true. With a little adjustment and imagination, healthful eating can actually be quite pleasant, just as it was for all those millions of years before the likes of the cream-filled Danish even appeared.

An optimally healthful diet will probably require a period of adjustment that involves some sacrifices, but when the deeper biological sense of what you're doing begins to kick in and the cravings developed over all those years of chips and dips begin to fade — and you start actually *feeling* better on the foods that give your body the essential nutrients it needs — you'll wonder how you ever got by on all those quasi foods in the first place. Some of what it takes to have a healthy diet can actually be enjoyable, in fact — things like eating as many meals a day as you want, making sure not to pass up those potatoes, and never letting yourself get hungry. By eating better, you'll actually enjoy eating *more*, because you'll be satisfying biological needs that go deeper than the frivolous taste buds on your tongue.

Please review the following guidelines with these perks in mind. And remember that food is more than just fuel. Most of your body's cells remanufacture themselves every few days, so what you eat, to a large degree, really does become part of you.

1. *Learn to look at fat as Dietary Demon No. 1.* The stuff has been implicated as a causative factor in heart disease, stroke, high blood pressure, and cancers of the colon, prostate, and breast. While surveys show we've been making progress against it (we're down from an average of 38 percent of calories to about 34 percent), we still have a way to go. The American Heart Association recommends about 30 percent, but some of the major health agencies would like us to strive for even lower than that — about 20 percent. Percentages are of little help when it comes to knowing how much fat you're actually putting on your

Foods Full of Fat

Next time you reach for the foods listed below, think again. By eating these foods sparingly, you'll be well on your way to a healthful low-fat diet based on this step alone.

FOOD	PERCENTAGE OF CALORIES FROM FAT
Cured meats such as hot dogs, sausage, salami, and bacon	about 80
Nuts	about 80
Hard cheeses	about 70
The more succulent cuts of beef and pork	about 60
Fried foods, such as chicken, fish, and french fries	about 60
Potato chips and other snack foods fried in oil	about 60
Full-fat dairy products such as whole milk and ice cream	about 50
Cookies, pastries, and pies	about 50

plate, but if you follow the rest of these guidelines, you should be within a safe 20 to 30 percent range.

2. Learn where fat lives. Fat is found in its most concentrated form in butter, margarine, cooking oils, and salad dressings, but it also resides in huge amounts in other foods (see "Foods Full of Fat" above).

3. Eat more fruits and vegetables. Rich in vital nutrients such as the antioxidant vitamins A and C, which help reduce risks of cancer, and potassium, which helps maintain healthy blood pressure, fruits and veggies also are great low-calorie, virtually fat-free sources of dietary fiber, needed to promote regularity and help protect against cancer of the colon.

4. Eat more potatoes, beans, rice, and bread. Again, high in nutrients (B vitamins, especially) and also fiber, these foods are low in calories and nearly free of fat. Combined properly, they can even be great fat-free sources of protein.

5. *Eat more fish.* Excellent sources of protein, most varieties of fish are very low in fat, and even those that aren't offer a type of fat (called omega-3 fatty acids) that actually seems to help protect against heart disease — and perhaps arthritis, as well.

6. *"Eat" more water.* And yes, do begin to think of water as a food. Chewable food, after all, we can do without for about 30 days; water, only about 3. All the very important biological reasons for that aside, taking in more water can be an aid to weight control because water fills us up with the lowest-calorie food on the planet. It also can be an energy booster by preventing chronic dehydration — a problem for all us "athletes" whose specialty is the rat race.

7. *Eat more frequently.* Now *here's* some music to your ears. Studies show not only that the body makes better use of the nutrients in food when it's eaten in smaller and more frequent amounts but also that calories are less likely to be converted to fat when we "graze" as opposed to gorge. The reason has to do with a blood component known as insulin, whose job it is to see that excess calories do not wander around dangerously in the bloodstream as glucose, but get used as energy or stored as fat instead. Since large meals mean a large insulin response, fat cells perk up, and, as a result, have a greater tendency to plump up on any calories *not* used for energy.

8. *Eat earlier in the day.* This means you should avoid that "I'm-so-busy-I-can-eat-only-at-night" syndrome. By taking in more of your calories during breakfast and lunch as opposed to dinner (and definitely as opposed to before bed) you accomplish two things: You give your body the food it needs *when* it needs it, thus fueling more energy mentally as well as physically; and you also avoid the heightened fat storage that happens when you sleep. Excess calories in the blood during periods of inactivity are more likely to be taken in by fat cells, studies show. When the body is active, on the other hand, muscle cells get first dibs on those potential fat-makers.

9. *Don't eat less until you've tried to eat better.* If you're overweight, it very well could be because of *what* you've been eating, not how much. This doesn't mean that calories don't count, because we know that they do. But when you eat foods high in calories and yet *low* in nutrients, your body cries out in protest until you have finally given it at least some semblance of what it needs. Put another way: There are a lot more body-pleasing nutrients in a breakfast of cottage cheese and whole-wheat toast than in a whole box of doughnuts.

10. Do not "diet." The word itself should serve as a warning (see below). The only "diet" that can work is the one you can stick to for the rest of your life.

The Folly of Dieting

What "dies" when people diet is the body's ability to do precisely what it *must* do if fat is going to be lost — burn calories. Dieting kills this crucial ability in three distinct ways:

■ *Dieting encourages the loss of the very instruments — muscle cells — that burn fat best.* Dieters may *think* they're losing only fat when they reduce their caloric intake, but studies show that muscle cells also get lost. This loss can be minimized if exercise is included as part of a low-calorie diet, but it can not be prevented entirely: The body always will "cannibalize" at least some muscle tissue when caloric intake is insufficient to meet the body's energy demands.

■ *Dieting robs the body of the energy it needs to burn fat correctly, which is through greater levels of physical activity.* Maybe you've experienced the syndrome yourself: After several days of lettuce and rice cakes you have all the get-up-and-go of a snail. Is that any way to burn calories? You bet it's not. As paradoxical as it may sound, burning fat requires taking in enough quality calories to give your body the energy it needs to do fat-burning exercise.

But perhaps most insidiously of all . . .

■ *Dieting makes what you do eat all the more fattening.* And isn't that the cruelest irony of all? By severely reducing caloric intake, you force your body into its evolutionarily acquired starvation mode, which lowers its calorie-burning rate. (Exercise, on the other hand, does just the opposite by setting into motion bio-chemical events that *speed* calorie burning.)

Eating healthfully is too time-consuming, you fear, not to mention *mind*-consuming? Counting calories was hard enough, but now there are grams of fat to worry about, and milligrams of sodium and cholesterol. That sort of vigilance can be tough, especially if you're the type to get antsy just waiting for a bacon double cheeseburger at the drive-up window of your local McDonald's.

If that's you, relax, take a deep breath, and repeat these words: "Eating healthfully can be a piece of cake. It can be easier and faster than eating *unhealthfully*, in fact, because there's less grease, fat, and fuss."

That's right. Healthful cooking and speedy cooking can go together like a knife and fork because the key to both is simplicity. It's those cream sauces and goose-liver pâtés that take time. You can poach up a piece of fish, "nuke" a potato, and steam some broccoli in less time than it would take to watch the evening news. Plus, you're not scrubbing a greasy skillet afterward, as you would by making an artery-clogging cheeseburger.

Better yet, speedier cooking can mean *better nutrition*, as research shows that less time in the oven or on the stove means fewer nutrients lost in the cooking process. The nutrients in fresh vegetables are especially sensitive, so by steaming your veggies for just a few minutes — or better yet, microwaving them — you avoid the absurdity of pouring the majority of their minerals and vitamins (vitamins A and C especially) down your kitchen sink.

But maybe best of all, healthful cooking can allow you, in many cases, to throw "portion control" to the wind. Make a really healthy vegetable-loaded stir-fry, for example, and you can pretty much serve yourself with a shovel. It's those well-marbled beef fillets you need to monitor by the nibble.

*Less time in the kitchen
can mean more health because
we're encouraged to cook quickly and simply.*

So please, no more excuses for not eating better because of too little time. It's when we *do* have time that we tend to tack on the fat and calories, as any respectable recipe from James or Julia will attest.

Breakfasts in a Fit (and Friendlier) Flash

You want to know the real reason we're often less civil than we'd like in the morning? Cite biorhythms, a bad night's sleep, or bad breath if you want to, but maybe it's also due to feeling rushed. We're usually just too *late* to be nice.

So why not add precious minutes to your morning madness with fast foods that are low in fat but high in protein and fiber, yet tasty enough to keep visions of glazed doughnuts from dancing through your head. Here are some dishes that can do just that:

The VIP "Porridge." Scoop together in a cereal bowl roughly equal parts of low-fat cottage cheese, your favorite flavored nonfat yogurt, wheat germ, dry oatmeal (optional), and a little skim milk. Add some orange juice for sweetness, and there's not a major nutrient this one doesn't have — in spades. Amazingly tasty as well.

The "Shake, Skedaddle, and Stroll." No blender (it's too hard to wash). Combine in a jar with a tight lid skim milk, low-fat vanilla yogurt, a couple of tablespoons of nonfat dry milk or protein powder (optional), and a splash of fruit juice (for more sweetness plus vitamin C). Shake like crazy. (Great for the pectoral muscles, biceps, triceps, forearms, and hands.)

The "Better Bagel." No more bagel abuse with the butter and the cream cheese. Keep your fat-free bagels innocent with this idea: a spread (made in bulk and kept in your refrigerator) consisting of plain low-fat yogurt combined with apple butter or whatever other jelly or marmalade you'd prefer. Warm the bagel slightly, spread with the mixture, and sprinkle with cinnamon or nutmeg.

An Eggselent Omelette. If you've not tried the egg substitutes (essentially eggs without the yolks), you should. Try an omelette with cottage cheese, low-fat mozzarella, and a splash of soy sauce made in a good, nonstick skillet.

Your Own Granola. Why buy the packaged stuff that may be packed with fat? Make your own, using raisins, oatmeal, wheat germ, and a high-vitamin cereal (such as Total or Product 19). With skim or low-fat milk, it's another nutritional gold mine.

Power-Packed Lunches with 500 or Fewer Calories

Research indicates that it's better to eat earlier in the day, when calories are more likely to get burned for energy than to get stored as fat. Protein seems to be particularly energizing, especially midway through the day. It's a long biochemical story, but its conclusion is that protein helps promote alertness while carbohydrates are inclined to induce a more relaxed state.

Here, then, are some protein-packed ideas for quick, low-fat, tasty midday repasts. All can be enjoyed for a scant 500 calories at most.

A tuna sandwich, made with water-packed tuna and low-fat mayonnaise — or for even more protein, low-fat cottage cheese.

A scoop of cottage cheese atop a warm raisin bagel with a few sprinkles of cinnamon (great for breakfast, too).

A smoked sliced turkey sandwich, with tomato and mustard.

An egg-substitute omelette, spiked with cottage cheese and canned mushrooms.

Also consider one of the hearty low-fat soups commercially available, or put one of the new low-fat cheeses, whole-grain crackers, and a piece of fresh fruit in your lunch bag. Half a chicken breast left over from a recent dinner and some hearty European-style bread make a simple, satisfying meal. And in a pinch, one of the high-protein, low-fat, vitamin-packed "shakes" can make a highly nutritious, if unmemorable, lunch.

The idea, remember, is to get plenty of energy-boosting protein into your midday meal, without the fat it frequently befriends.

If you're beginning to get the feeling that highly nutritional food can be just as fast to prepare as the "fast-food variety," you're right. No lines, that's for sure. Eating high on health requires just two steps, in fact.

#1	#2
Know the most healthful foods to cook:	Cook them in the most healthful ways:
Fish	bake, broil, grill, poach
Chicken	bake, roast, grill
Lean cuts of beef and pork	broil, grill
Vegetables	microwave, steam, blanch
Potatoes	bake, boil, microwave
Beans	boil
Rice	boil
Fruits	are best eaten raw

Fast and Healthy Dinner Ideas

After a killer day, the last thing you're in the mood for is playing Julia Child, so here are some ideas for low-fat, highly nutritious "quickies" that Julia herself might actually enjoy.

Stir-fry, using *plenty* of fresh vegetables. It can help tremendously to have a high-quality, nonstick skillet or wok when stir-frying so that you'll use as little oil as possible — preferably no more than about a tablespoon, recommends the master of low-fat cuisine Graham Kerr. For your protein source, chicken and shrimp are lowest in fat, but lean cuts of beef and pork are fair game, too.

Hearty low-fat soups and stews. Prepare them in advance; weekends are a good time for cooking. Make enough for several dinners, and refrigerate or freeze the surplus. Accompanied by some fresh whole-grain bread and a salad, soups and stews are extremely healthful, and lightning quick to heat up.

Pasta dishes. They don't take much longer than boiling water, and with all the fantastic, low-fat sauces now available, you can have your taste of Italy and size 6, too.

Slow-cooker meals. You've seen them and maybe you even have one — those large, covered electrically powered kettles that cook pretty much on their own while you work or are otherwise occupied. You simply load one up, set its timer for when you want to eat, and bingo: Dinner is ready when you are. Great for chicken, beef, pork roasts, and especially stews.

Broiled fish. Possibly the most healthful quick dinner of all. Serve it with a microwaved potato or rice and some steamed or microwaved veggies — and your heart will thank you.

HUNGER: RESPECT IT, DON'T REJECT IT

And finally, a word on hunger — that Waterloo of weight loss that is perhaps the greatest impediment of all to our fat-fighting efforts. Our mistake, believe it or not, is that we usually attempt to defy our hunger when we would be far wiser, studies show, to comply with it.

This isn't to say you should instantaneously surrender to every craving that may come your way, but it does mean you should eat when your body signals that it's legitimately hungry. To ignore these signals is to allow your body to believe it's in the throes of a famine, to which it will respond by storing what few calories you *do* consume as fat rather than making them readily available to your muscles to be burned for energy. Worse yet, your body will begin to actually metabolize muscle tissue for energy if you let your food intake drop too low — and your muscles, of course, are the best fat-burners you have.

So please don't foil your weight-control efforts — or your exercise efforts, either — by failing to give your body the energy it needs to succeed at both of these pursuits. Keep reminding yourself that it takes energy to burn fat, because it takes energy to be physically active. What better reason to keep yourself well stoked with healthful foods than that?

1. Eat more fruits and vegetables – 2 fruits + 1 vegetable daily

2. Eat only 1 cup of cereal in the morning

3. Substitute other snacks for chips = baked chips vegetables

4. Make a list of other activities to do instead of "stress-relief eating"

Oakland County Health Division

1200 N. Telegraph Rd.
Pontiac, MI 48341-1043
(248) 858-1280
Toll Free 1-888-350-0900

1010 E. West Maple Rd.
Walled Lake, MI 48390-3588
(248) 926-3300

Contact us at our Website:
www.co.oakland.mi.us

27725 Greenfield Rd.
Southfield, MI 48076-3625
(248) 424-7000

54 • HENS • N 607 • 5-98

THE EXERCISES

Exercise can be incorporated into everything we do, but it's important to do the right *kind* of exercises and to do them correctly. Exercising incorrectly can add to stress rather than relieve it, since very few benefits are gained, and time is lost. View the following exercises with that in mind. Done consistently and correctly, they can be the foundation of fitness success.

STRETCHES TO DO ANYWHERE

If you're confined to one place for hours at a time at an office, in a classroom, at a counter, or at home, working stretches into your day can help you avoid stiffness in addition to keeping you energized enough to be at your best.

SHOULDER ROTATIONS

This simple maneuver can loosen tight shoulders caused by pro-longed periods of sitting.

1. While taking deep, slow breaths, move the tip of one shoulder in a large circular pattern for about one minute, changing direction midway. Let the movement be as smooth as possible.

2. Repeat with the other shoulder.

UPPER BACK STRETCH

This stretch targets the muscles of the shoulders and upper back to ease the stiffness caused by sitting.

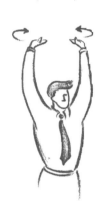

1. While sitting or standing, stretch your arms upward and slightly behind you (as if you were a football referee signaling a touchdown). Take a deep breath and exhale.

2. With palms facing the ceiling, rotate your thumbs forward as far as they will go and take another deep breath.

3. Repeat whenever needed.

UPPER BACK SQUEEZE

Do this quick and easy movement wherever you are throughout the day.

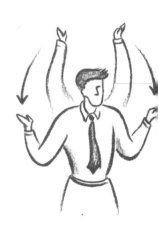

1. While sitting or standing, raise your arms above your head and stretch, taking a deep breath.

2. Exhale as you lower your elbows behind you as low as you can, pressing your shoulder blades together and keeping your palms facing upward. Keep your back and neck still throughout the movement.

3. Hold for 10 seconds then return to starting position and repeat 3 times.

NECK STRETCH

This is another godsend for those who must sit for long periods of time, especially in front of a computer. It's ideal for relieving stiffness in the neck and increasing range of motion.

1. With your left hand behind your lower back, place the palm of your right hand on the back of your head.

2. Tucking your chin gently, slowly pull your head forward and downward as far as is comfortable. Hold for 5 seconds, taking a deep breath in and out.

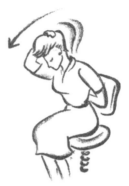

3. Return your arms to your sides and keep your chin tucked gently. With your face forward, bend your head toward your right shoulder. (Keep your shoulder relaxed.) Hold for 5 seconds, taking a deep breath in and out.

4. Now repeat #1 and #2 with your right hand behind your lower back and the palm of your left hand on the back of your head.

5. Repeat #3, moving your head to the left.

CHIN TUCK

Just what the doctor ordered to melt away stiffness in the neck, chest, and shoulders. Do this exercise several times a day. Over time, it may actually help stretch tight tissues and lengthen the neck.

1. While sitting or standing upright, slowly move your erect head to the rear, keeping your nose pointed straight ahead, until you feel a gentle stretch in the back of your head and neck. (You're doing it correctly if you suddenly develop a double chin.)

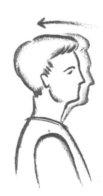

2. Hold this position for 5 seconds, then repeat for a total of 3 times.

SHOULDER STRETCH

Put this one on your list of stretches to ease the stress of sitting, too.

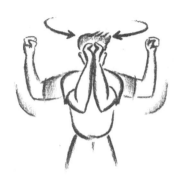

1. While sitting or standing, raise your arms with elbows bent until upper arms are parallel to the floor. Squeeze your shoulder blades together and take a deep breath in and out. Relax.

2. Slowly bring your arms together in front of you, your elbows touching if possible. Take a deep breath in and out.

3. Repeat for a total of 3 times.

LOWER BACK STRETCH

This stretch is good for squeezing the tension out of an aching lower back. Do this after bending over a desk or work area for extended periods.

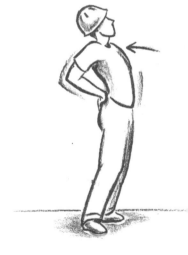

1. While standing or sitting, place your palms on your lower back and lean backward. Hold for a count of 5, then straighten back up.

2. Repeat for a total of 3 times.

TORSO TWISTER

Good for loosening tight muscles of the neck, back, and hips.

1. While sitting with your feet apart and flat on the floor, rotate your torso to one side, keeping your chin tucked and your knees pointed straight ahead. Breath in and out.

2. Turn to the opposite side and repeat for a total of 3 times to each side.

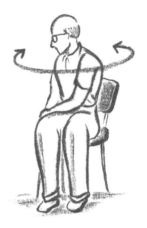

HIP SWITCH WITH NECK STRETCH

When you have to stay seated for more than half an hour, this simple stretch will be a welcome relief.

1. While sitting, lean to one side so that your weight rests on one hip. Keeping your chin tucked, turn your head to the opposite side. Take a deep breath in and out.

2. Repeat for a total of 3 times in each direction.

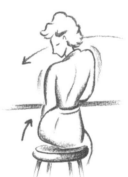

STRETCHES TO DO AT HOME

Simply stretching out on the floor can bring relief to a tired body. But there's much more you can do while relaxing at home to de-stress your muscles and become more flexible.

THE BACK BENDER

This can bring welcome relief to stiffness in the lower back after a long day of sitting — or getting stuck in traffic on your way home.

1. Lie on your stomach with your hands in front of your face.

2. Slowly, gently straighten your arms to press your upper body off the floor while your hips and lower body remain stationary. Straighten until you feel a gentle stretch in your lower back.

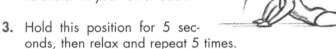

3. Hold this position for 5 seconds, then relax and repeat 5 times.

HAMSTRING STRETCH

This is another great stretch for those of us who sit for long periods. It's also a good stretch to complement a running or walking program because it can help prevent injury to the hamstrings. It can also help prevent lower back pain.

1. With a pillow under your head, lie on the floor in a doorway.

2. Raise one leg so that your heel rests against the door jamb and you begin to feel a stretching sensation in the muscles at the back of your thigh. (The straighter you can keep your leg, the better, but go slowly if you cannot straighten your leg completely.)

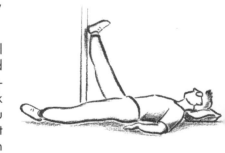

3. Hold this position for about 20 seconds, then switch to the other leg and repeat the sequence twice.

CALF STRETCH

This is a good stretch to do after running or walking, to keep the calves from becoming tight.

1. Position yourself facing a wall with your hands against it. Place one foot about two feet behind the other.

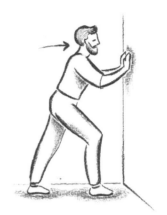

2. While keeping your back leg straight and both feet flat on the floor, bend your front leg until you feel a slight pulling sensation in the calf muscle of your rear leg. Make sure your back heel stays flat on the floor. Hold this position for about 30 seconds.

3. Repeat with the legs switched.

SIDE BENDS

This can help loosen the muscles of the "love handle" area, which can become tight after too many hours of being desk-bound.

1. Stand against a wall with your feet about a foot apart. Make sure your knees are not "locked" back.

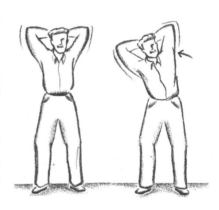

2. Clasp your hands over your head (or place your hands on your hips if that's more comfortable) and slowly bend as far as you can to one side, keeping your head, shoulders, and buttocks against the wall for support. Hold the stretch in the bent position for up to 30 seconds.

3. Repeat, bending to the other side. Do for a total of 2 times to each side, breathing deeply.

THE HIP AND THIGH STRETCHER

This maneuver can help keep the muscles at the front of the thigh (the quadriceps) limber as well as the muscles that control movement in the hips.

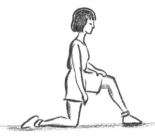

1. Kneel on the floor and bring one leg forward with foot on the floor and knee bent.

2. Tighten your abdominal muscles and lean forward (without arching your back) so that you begin to feel the stretch at the front of your thigh. For proper alignment, keep your bent front knee over your foot.

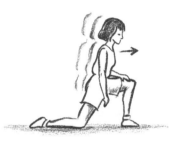

3. Hold this position for 20 seconds, then switch legs and repeat twice.

THE BUTT STRETCHER

Here's one tailor-made for frequent sitters. It helps to loosen muscles in the area of the buttocks and hips.

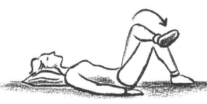

1. Lie on your back with a pillow behind your head and place one foot so that it rests on your opposite knee.

2. Reaching through your legs, use both hands to grasp the leg that's serving as a prop, and gently pull it toward your chest. (Use a towel to help you do this, if you wish.) Feel the stretch in your buttocks.

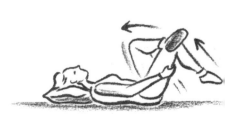

3. Hold this position for 20 seconds, then switch legs and repeat twice.

THE JACKKNIFE

Consider this one a staple. It can do a great job of alleviating low back pain by stretching the muscles of both the lower back and the thighs.

1. Lie on your back with one leg bent at approximately a 90° angle and the foot of that leg flat on the floor.

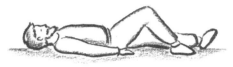

2. Grasp the knee of the bent leg from behind and pull it into your chest while keeping your other leg straight and in full contact with the floor.

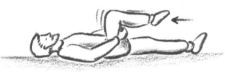

3. Hold this position for 20 seconds, then switch legs and repeat as often as feels comfortable.

THE QUADRI-STRETCH

Good for loosening the quadriceps, the muscles at the front of the thigh.

1. Lying on your side, keep your thighs together as you pull the heel of the top leg toward your buttocks until you feel a comfortable stretch. Keep your back straight and don't let it arch. (If you can't reach your foot with your hand, use a tie or a sock around your ankle.)

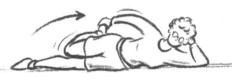

2. Hold for 20 seconds, switch legs, and repeat.

Variation

You can also do the Quadri-Stretch while standing by bracing yourself with your hand against a wall.

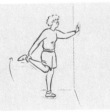

STRENGTH-BUILDING EXERCISES

Good muscle tone depends on frequent muscle use, but who gets to do much of that in our high-tech world? You can, even if your job is a totally sedentary one. You can do these exercises anywhere, anytime, and *without* any equipment.

ARM CIRCLES

Important for maintaining good range of motion in the shoulders and strengthening arm muscles, this exercise can be done even while sitting at your desk. (Try doing it in the rest room if you're concerned that co-workers may think you've flipped your lid.)

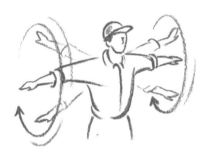

1. Stand or sit with your arms held straight out from your sides.

2. Begin moving your arms in circles, starting with small ones and getting larger as you go, for a period of 30 seconds.

3. Rest, then repeat 3 times.

ISOMETRIC CURLS

Here's a great way to firm and strengthen the biceps, forearms, triceps, and pectorals (chest muscles) all at once — and without anyone knowing what you're doing! Do these standing, sitting, or reclining.

1. With your elbows bent at 90° angles, turn your left forearm so that the palm of your left hand is facing up. Now place the palm of your right hand over the wrist of your upturned left arm.

2. Lift upward with your left hand with all the force you can muster, and at the same time press downward with your right. Your hands will remain essentially stationary. Hold for about 5 seconds.

3. Relax for about 10 seconds, then repeat 3 or 4 times. Switch hands and repeat 4 or 5 times.

CHAIR DIPS

This is a wonderful exercise for firming the triceps (the muscles at the back of the arm) plus the pectorals (the muscles of the chest). You can do dips using any chair that has arms.

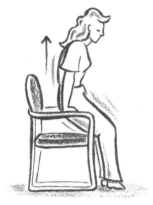

1. Place your palms on the arms of the chair and extend your arms until they are straight, lifting yourself off the chair.

2. Hold for a second or longer, then slowly lower yourself until you're sitting.

3. Repeat up to 5 times.

DESK DIPS

Dips can also be done using the edge of any desk or countertop sturdy enough to support you.

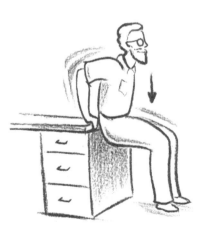

1. Stand with your back to the desk or countertop and your feet 6 to 12 inches in front of it. Bend your knees as much as you need to, position your hands on the edge of the desk behind you, palms down, arms straight.

2. Using the muscles of your arms, lower yourself slowly as far as is comfortable.

3. Slowly press yourself back up until your arms are straight. Repeat as many times as you can.

THE PRAYER

This is another great way to firm the muscles of the chest, but it also does a nice job of working the "lats" (latissimus dorsi muscles) of the back. Do it at your desk, while waiting in line at the supermarket, or any other time you have a few minutes to kill.

1. Place your palms together in front of your chest.

2. Press your hands together as hard as you can. (Your elbows will come up as you do.)

3. Hold for 5 seconds, relax for 10 seconds, and repeat 5 times or until tired.

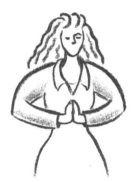

DOORWAY DELTOID STRENGTHENER

This is a back-handed version of the maneuver Samson used to "bring down the house" on the Philistines. Do it to build up the deltoids, the muscles at the tips of the shoulders.

1. Stand in a doorway with your arms straight down at your sides, palms in, and move your arms out from your sides until the backs of your hands meet the doorjamb.

2. Keeping your arms straight, try to raise them, pressing against the doorjamb, with all the force you can.

3. Continue this exertion for about 5 seconds, relax for 10 seconds, then repeat 4 more times.

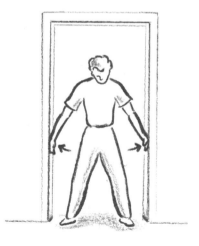

SHOULDER PUSH

Good for strengthening the scapular muscles (around the shoulder blades). This also can be done with whatever weights you may have available.

1. Lying on your back, grasp a 1-pound weight in each hand and hold them near your chest.

2. Keeping your back against the floor, push the weights up toward the ceiling until your arms are straight.

3. Hold for 5 seconds. Repeat for a total of 10.

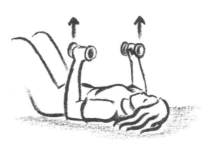

THE BUTTERFLY

If your shoulders feel tight, this exercise will feel great and also help strengthen them.

1. Grasping a 1-pound weight in each hand, lie facedown with your forehead against the floor. (If you are too uncomfortable, turn you head to the side. There shouldn't be any strain on the neck, though.)

2. Holding your arms out from your shoulders and keeping your elbows bent, squeeze your shoulder blades together.

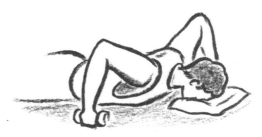

3. Hold for 1 second. Repeat for a set of 10.

As your shoulder and arm strength improves, challenge yourself by increasing the number of sets you perform and the size of your weights. Use canned goods if you don't want to invest in exercise equipment.

- After you can easily do a single set of 10, progress to 2 sets of 10 and then 3 sets of 10.
- When you can easily do 3 sets of 10, start using 2½-pound hand weights for a single set of 10.
- Increase to 2 sets of 10 using the 2½-pound weights; then to 3 sets.
- When you are comfortable doing 3 sets with the 2½-pound weights, begin with a single set using 5-pound weights.
- Increase the sets as you are ready.

Your arms should feel tired after your workout but for no more than several hours. If the exercises are painful or you are very sore after doing them, decrease the number of repetitions and/or the size of the weights. You're ready to progress when the workout becomes easy.

SUPERMAN
Another good shoulder stretcher and strengthener, this maneuver can be done in bed as well as on the floor.

1. Lying facedown and holding 1-pound weights in each hand, stretch your arms straight out above your head. Keep your forehead on the floor.

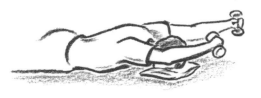

2. Raise your arms from the floor and hold for 5 seconds. Relax.

3. Repeat for a set of 10.

CHEST FLIES

Your shoulder muscles and pectorals (chest muscles) will benefit from this exercise.

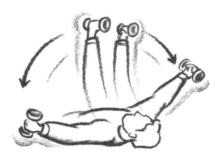

1. Holding a 1-pound weight in each hand, lie on your back and stretch your arms out straight to each side on the floor.

2. Slowly raise both arms at the same time until your hands meet. Bring them slowly back down again.

3. Repeat for a set of 10.

STANDING LIFTS

This exercise is another good one for strengthening arms and shoulders.

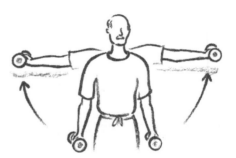

1. Holding 1-pound weights, stand straight with arms at your sides.

2. Slowly raise your arms out from your body to each side, hold briefly, and then slowly lower.

3. Repeat for a set of 10.

STANDING BACK LIFTS

For strong, flexible shoulders and upper back, do this maneuver whenever you can spare a few minutes.

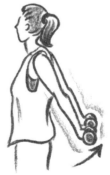

1. Stand straight while holding a 1-pound weight in each hand.

2. Slowly raise your arms up and backward while keeping your elbows straight. Hold briefly, and slowly lower.

3. Repeat for a set of 10.

SEMI SIT-UPS

This is a good tummy-tightener, effective for firming the "abs" but also for preventing low back pain by strengthening muscles responsible for supporting the spine.

1. Lie on your back with your legs bent at a 90° angle. Keeping your chin tucked, slowly raise your head and shoulders off the floor.

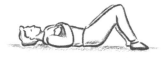

2. Hold this position for 5 seconds, slowly lie back down, and repeat 10 times.

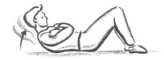

3. Following the same procedure as above, raise your head and shoulders to the right 10 times. Repeat 10 times to the left.

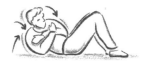

Caution: Make sure that your neck stays relaxed. The power should come from your abs.

3 STYLES OF SEMI SIT-UPS

Modify these sit-ups to work with your level of fitness.

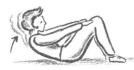
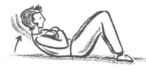
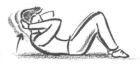

Beginning exercisers should extend arms straight out in front.

Intermediate exercisers should fold their arms across their chest.

Advanced exercisers should place their hands behind their necks.

THE LOWER AB BUILDER

This exercise helps firm the lower abdominal region, that area some-times unflatteringly called the "paunch."

1. Begin by lying on the floor with your knees bent and your feet flat on the floor, your arms at your sides.

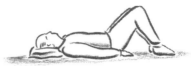

2. Lift your knees toward your stomach and begin a pedaling action.

3. Continue for 10 seconds, rest, and repeat several more times.

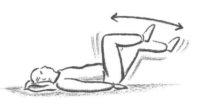

Caution: Make sure your neck stays relaxed. The power should come from your abs.

PELVIC TILT

This is a great exercise that you can do almost anywhere to strength-en the muscles of your abdomen.

1. While standing or sitting, tighten your stomach muscles as you curl your buttocks forward.

2. Hold for a count of 5 and repeat at least 3 times.

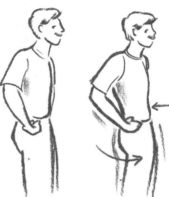

THE BACK AND BUTT BUILDER

This exercise is a real workhorse, simultaneously strengthening the muscles of the hamstrings, buttocks, and abdominals as it also strengthens the lower back.

1. Lie facedown with your feet slightly apart and your arms stretched out in front of you.

2. While keeping your head down and your abdominal muscles tightened, lift one leg and the opposite arm 3 to 6 inches off the floor.

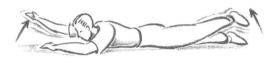

3. Hold this position for at least 1 second. Repeat 10 times, then switch to your other leg and arm.

THE WALL SLIDE

This is a dynamite way to firm and strengthen the upper thighs.

1. Stand with your back against a wall.

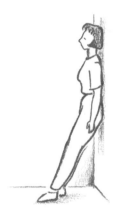

2. Move your feet out from the wall about a foot. Slide your body down along the wall until your knees are bent at approximately a 45° angle.

3. Hold for a count of 10, then press back up.

4. Repeat 10 times or until tired.

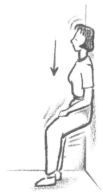

THE QUADRIPED

This is an excellent exercise for lumbar stabilization: preventing low back pain by strengthening the muscles responsible for supporting the lower (lumbar) region of the spine. In this case, the buttocks muscles are targeted.

1. Begin by getting down on all fours.

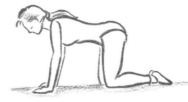

2. Keeping your hips level, extend your left leg behind you until it's parallel to the floor.

3. Hold for at least 1 second, repeat 10 times, then do the same with your right leg.

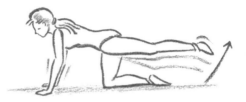

Caution: Keep your back flat to prevent lumbar compression and to make sure you are using the correct muscles.

Variation

For an even tougher version, try extending your leg and opposite arm simultaneously.

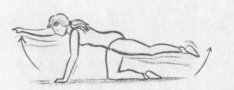

LEG RAISES

These exercises strengthen the quadriceps and also are good for the hips and knees.

1. Sitting with hands slightly behind you on the floor, extend one leg and bend the other. Pull the toes of the straight leg toward you and press the back of the knee down.

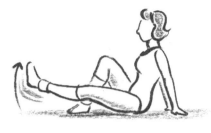

2. Raise the straight leg 6 to 8 inches, then slowly lower it to the floor. Relax. Repeat for a set of 10.

3. Do the same with the other leg for a set of 10.

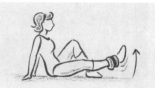

Variation

Add ankle weights once leg raises become effortless.

SIDE LEG RAISES

This exercise is great for firming the muscles of the upper thigh, which when flabby can resemble saddlebags.

1. Lie on one side, propping your head on one hand and using the other hand in front of you for support.

2. Slowly raise your top leg as far as you comfortably can, hold for at least 5 seconds, and lower slowly and steadily. Repeat for a set of 10.

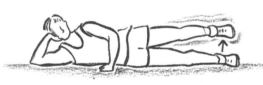

3. Switch sides. Do the side leg raises with the other leg for a set of 10.

Caution: Make sure your hips stay perpendicular to the floor and don't roll forward or backward.

As your leg muscles grow stronger after doing these exercises consistently over a period of time, increase the number of sets you do and add weights. Use this progression and you'll see a big improvement.

- When you can do 1 set of 10 easily, start doing 2 sets of 10.
- When 2 sets becomes easy for you, increase your workout to 3 sets of 10.
- When you can do 3 sets of 10, add 1-pound ankle weights and decrease the repetitions to 1 set.
- Work up from 1 set of 10 with the weights to 3 sets.
- When you can easily do 3 sets with the 1-pound weights, move on to 2½-pound weights. Decrease the sets and work up to 3 again.
- Go to 5-pound weights when you've mastered the 2½-pound weights.

BACK LEG RAISES

This variation of the leg raise targets the back thigh and buttocks muscles.

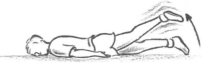

1. Lying on your stomach, slowly raise one leg as far as you comfortably can. Hold for 5 seconds and slowly lower.

2. Complete a set of 10 and repeat with the other leg.

INNER LEG RAISES

The adductor muscles on the inside of your upper leg are often neglected through disuse. This simple exercise will strengthen them.

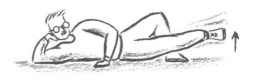

1. Lying on your side, bend your top leg behind the other. Propping yourself with your hand in front of you, raise your straight leg up.

2. Hold for at least 1 second and then lower slowly. Repeat for a set of 10. Switch sides and repeat.

Caution: Make sure your hips stay perpendicular to the floor and don't roll forward or backward.

TOE RAISES

Here's a great way to firm the calves. You can do these while working in the kitchen or even while standing in one of those lines modern life seems so good at putting in front of us.

1. Raise both heels from the floor until you are standing on your toes. Use a countertop or wall to help support you if balance becomes a problem.

2. Lower slowly and repeat 10 times (or as often as is appropriate for the line you're waiting in).

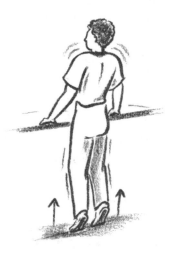

THE HIP FIRMER

Here's a way to help firm the muscles of the hip area that you can do even while watching TV.

1. Sit with your back straight and your arms at your sides.

2. Slowly lift your right knee up toward your chest (being sure to keep your back straight) as you push downward on your knee with your right arm to provide additional resistance.

3. Hold this position for about 3 seconds, repeat 3 times and repeat the procedure with your left leg and arm.

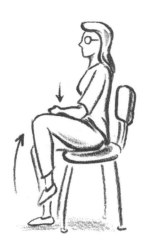

INSTANT STRESS-BUSTERS

Stress takes its toll on muscles by keeping them in a contract-ed state. One of the best ways of combating the physical effects of stress, therefore, is to stretch these tightened muscles to help them relax. Another benefit of stretching is the wonderful way it makes you feel, physically and mentally. Could it be that the physical flexibility that results from stretching is mirrored by a more flexible state of mind? With more and more being dis-covered about the mind-body connection, it's not unreasonable to speculate!

THE SHOULDER SHRUG

Slowly raise your shoulders toward your ears and hold for 10 seconds while inhal-ing and exhaling deeply. Relax, and repeat 3 times.

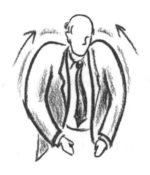

THE SURRENDER SQUEEZE

Raise your hands slightly above your shoulders, move your elbows backward to squeeze your shoulder blades together, and hold for 10 seconds while inhaling and exhaling. Relax, and repeat 3 times.

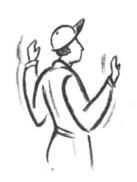

THE NECK EXTENDER

Pretend a cable is attached to the top of your head, extend your neck upward as if the cable were pulling you, and hold for 10 seconds while breathing deeply. Relax, and repeat 3 times.

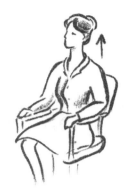

THE SHAKE

While standing or sitting, drop your arms to your sides and gently begin to shake your hands, feeling the tension leave as you do.

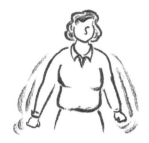

THE REACH

While sitting or standing, extend your arms as high as possible over your head, and hold for 5 seconds as you breathe deeply. Relax, and repeat 5 times.

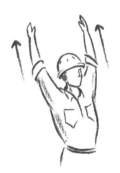

THE SHOULDER ROLL

Using a wide circular motion, roll your shoulders backward for about 30 seconds.

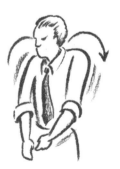

Other Publications for Boosting Health

BOOKS

Alexander, Tania, and Andy Jackson. *The Fitkid Adventure Book: Health-Related Fitness for 5 to 14 Year Olds*. North Pomfret, VT: Trafalgar Square, 1995.

Arnot, Robert. *Dr. Bob Arnot's Guide to Turning Back the Clock, Vol. I: A Complete Fitness Program for Men*. Boston, MA: Little, Brown & Company, 1995.

Brown, Marguerite. *Born to Be Fit: Discover Your Natural Ability to Be Happy, Healthy & Fit*. Lockport, NY: Tell Publishing, 1996.

Burke, Edmund B., editor. *Complete Home Fitness Handbook*. Champaign, IL: Human Kinetics Publisher, 1995.

Butler, Joan M. *Fit & Pregnant: The Pregnant Woman's Guide to Exercise*. Waverly, NY: Acorn Publishing, 1996.

Dauphinee, Rosanne C. *Eat Well & Live Cookbook*. Patten, ME: Majestic House Press, 1995.

Ettinger, Walter H., Brenda Mitchell, and Steven N. Blair. *Fitness After 50: It's Never Too Late to Start*. Maryland Heights, MO: Beverly Cracom Publications, 1996.

Fit to be Tried: A Program for Lifetime Fitness. Clearwater, FL: Lindsay Press, 1996.

Gaut, Ed. *The Joy of Fitness*. Minocqua, WI: Willow Creek Publications, 1996.

Graham, Gregg, Chip Blasium, and Ralfie Blasium. *Fun Fitness for Young Bodies*. Fort Wayne, IN: B.C. Creations, 1996.

Harrison, James C. *Hooked on Fitness! Fun Physical Conditioning Games & Activities*. Indianapolis, IN: Prentice Hall, 1996.

Hawkins, Jerald D., and Sandra M. Hawkins. *Walking for Fun & Fitness*. Englewood, CO: Morton Publishing Company, 1996.

Heady, Robert K. *Complete Idiot's Guide to Getting & Keeping Your Perfect Body*. Indianapolis, IN: Macmillan Publishing Company, Inc., 1996.

Hoffman, Lisa, and Anita W. Bell. *The Midlife Woman's Workout Program*. Boston, MA: Houghton Mifflin Company, 1996.

Jackowski, Edward. *Hold It! You're Exercising Wrong: Your Prescription for First-Class Fitness — Fast!* Indianapolis, IN: Simon & Schuster, 1995.

Jacobs, Miriam. *The 10% Low-Fat Cookbook: 200 Tantalizing Recipes with No More Than 10% Calories from Fat*. Pownal, VT: Storey Publishing, 1997.

Lawler, Susan, and Katherine Graham. *Moms on the Move: The Complete Fitness Guide for Pregnancy & Postpartum*. Studio City, CA: Logan House Publications, 1996.

Lutter, Judy, and Lynn Jaffee. *The Bodywise Woman*. Champaign, IL: Human Kinetics Publishers, 1996.

Merker, Kyle. *The Fitness Guide: Where to Work Out When You're on the Road*. New York, NY: Incline Press Publishing, 1996.

Myers, H. Ann. *Fifty Ways to Leave Your Love Handles: Your Guide to Healthier Eating & More Enjoyable Exercise in 50 Quick Tips*. Denver, CO: Fresh Aer Health & Fitness, Inc., 1995.

Oh, Dr. *Fitness for the Busy Executive in Only Ten Minutes a Day: A Lifetime Program to Stay in Shape for Your Best Top Level Performance (Life Management Series)*. Solana Beach, CA: Better Life Books, 1996.

Pace, Adele, and Maria Jones. *The Busy Executive's Guide to Total Fitness*. Indianapolis, IN: Prentice Hall, 1995.

Paffenbarger, Ralph, and Eric Olsen. *LifeFit*. Champaign, IL: Human Kinetics Publishers, 1996.

Peters, Jean M., and Howard K. Peters Jr. *The Flexibility Manual*. Berwyn, PA: Sports Kinetics, Inc., 1995.

Ryan, E. Davis, and Charles Swencionis, Ph.D. *The Lazy Person's Guide to Fitness*. New York, NY: Barricade Books, Inc., 1994.

Samuelson, Joan B., and Gloria Averbuch. *Joan Benoit Samuelson's Running for Women*. Emmaus, PA: Rodale Press, 1995.

Smith, Kathy, and Susan Schlosberg. *Kathy Smith's Fitness Makeover: A 10-Week Guide to Exercise & Nutrition That Will Change Your Life*. New York, NY: Warner Books, Inc., 1997

Stamford, Bryant A., and Becca Coffin. *The Jack Sprat Low-Fat Diet: A Twenty Eight-Day, Heart-Healthy Plan You Can Follow the Rest of Your Life*. Lexington, KY: University Press of Kentucky, 1995.

Stanford Center for Research in Disease Prevention Staff. *Fresh Start: The Stanford Medical School Whole-Life Health & Fitness Program*. San Francisco, CA: KQED Books, 1996.

Weider, Joe, and Men's Fitness Magazine Staff. *Men's Fitness Magazine's Complete Guide to Health & Well-Being: The Ultimate Sourcebook for Men's Physical & Emotional Needs*. New York, NY: HarperCollins Publishers, Inc., 1996.

MAGAZINES

American Health (general health); Retirement Living Publishing Co., Inc.: New York, NY.

Bicycling (cycling, plus general health and fitness); Rodale Press: Emmaus, PA.

Health (general health); Hippocrates Partners: San Francisco, CA.

Heart & Soul (general health for African-Americans); Rodale Press: Emmaus, PA.

Men's Health (fitness and health for men); Rodale Press: Emmaus, PA.

Prevention (general health); Rodale Press: Emmaus, PA.

Shape Magazine (fitness and health for women); Weider Publications: Woodland Hills, CA.

Runner's World (running, plus general fitness and health); Rodale Press: Emmaus, PA.

The Walking Magazine (walking, plus general fitness and health); Walking, Inc.: Boston, MA.

Health and Fitness Information

Aerobics and Fitness Association of America
Fitness Advice Hotline
800-YOUR-BODY
Only the first 3 minutes are free.

American Council on Exercise
5820 Oberlin Drive, Suite 102
San Diego, CA 92121-3787
Consumer Fitness Hotline:
800-529-8227

Consumer Nutrition Hotline
American Dietetic Association
800-366-1655

National Federation of Professional Trainers
P.O. Box 4579
Lafayette, IN 47903
317-447-3296
800-729-6378
http://www.nfpt.com/nfpt

National Health Information Center
P.O. Box 1133
Washington, DC 20013-1133
800-336-4797
email: nhicinfo@health.org
http://nhic-nt.health.org

Nordic Track Health and Fitness Information Center
103 Peazy Road
Chaska, MN 55318
800-358-3636

The President's Council on Physical Fitness and Sports
701 Pennsylvania Avenue, NW
Washington, DC 20004-2608
202-272-3421

Note: Page numbers in italics denote illustrations.

Jefferson, Thomas, 115
Jogging, 37, 41, 59, 97, 101, 110
  calories burned by, 63, 102
Journal of the American Medical Association, 8, 13
Jumping jacks, 40, 46, 50, 89, 100
Jumping rope, 40, 41, 43, 82, 90, 93, 100
Kerr, Graham, 135
Kostrubala, Thaddeus, 87–88
Kun, Paula K., 81
Lack of exercise, 1–4
  dangers of, 13
LaLanne, Jack, 5, 29–30
Lee, Pamela, 120
Leg lifts, 27
Leg Raises, 156, *156*
Lincoln, Abraham, 115
Long Stretch, 38
Lower Ab Builder, 153, *153*
Lower Back Stretch, 51, 140, *140*
Lunches, 134
Lunchtime exercising, 57–59
Maximum heart rate, 26
Maxwell, Carolyn, 68
Moreno, Rita, 65
Morning exercises, 35–46
Mowing grass, 9, 27, 74, 75
Murray, Arthur, 64–65
Muscles, importance of, 27–29
National Association for Sport and Physical Education, 81
National Cancer Institute, 128
National Center for Health Statistics (NCHS), 6
Neck Extender, 160, *160*
Neck pain, 30
Neck Stretch, 42, 51, 139, *139*
New England Journal of Medicine, 11–12
Nicotine, 111
Nietzsche, Friedrich, 115
Non-desk workers, exercise for, 56–57
Nureyev, Rudolf, 65
Obesity, 6, 80
Osteoporosis, 14, 127
Pelvic Tilt, 153, *153*
Performance Edge, The (Robert K. Cooper), 16, 46
Ping-Pong (table tennis), 9, 107
Playground/playgym, 83–84

Podell, Ronald, 79
Prayer (exercise), 95, 148, *148*
President's Council on Physical Fitness and Sports, 7
Prevention magazine, 108
Prevention Walking Club, 108
Prowse, Juliet, 65
Pull-ups, 27
Push-ups, 27, 30, 31, 36, 97, 100
  wall, 50
Quadriped, 51, 155, *155*
Quadri-Stretch, 145, *145*
Racquetball, 64, 107
Raking leaves, 27, 75, 76
Reach, 51, 160, *160*
Reaching, 27
Reece, Gabrielle, 104
Rippe, James, 112
Rowing, 36, 40, 50, 59, 117, 119
Running, 27, 31, 37, 41, 101–3, 114, 127
  calories burned by, 63, 102
  in place, 40, 50, 97, 99, 100
  treadmill, 40, 50
Schwarzenegger, Arnold, 29, 97, 120
Scott, Warren, 8, 10, 23–24
Scuba diving, 107
Semi Sit-ups, 44, 100, 152, *152*
Sexual vigor, 111
Shake, 160, *160*
Shorter exercise segments, benefits of, 20–21, 23–24
Shoulder pain, 30
Shoulder Push, 149, *149*
Shoulder Roll, 57, 99, 160, *160*
Shoulder Rotations, 39, 42, 47, 51, 137, *137*
Shoulder Shrug, 99, 159, *159*
Shoulder Stretch, 42, 140, *140*
Side Bends, 143, *143*
Side Leg Raises, 156, *156*
Simmons, Richard, 13
Sitting
  calories burned by, 63
  lessons on, 54
Sit-ups, 27, 31, 94–95, 99
  Semi, 44, 100, 152, *152*
Skateboarding, 82
Skating, 37
  ice, 63
  in-line, 66, 82, 107
  roller, 63